W0050777

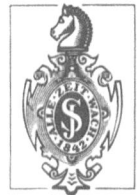

Judy Moyes · V. Ralph McCready · Ann Fullbrook

Neuroblastoma
mIBG in its Diagnosis and Management

With 241 Figures

Springer-Verlag
London Berlin Heidelberg New York
Paris Tokyo

Judy S. E. Moyes, MA (Cantab), FRCP (C)
Honorary Senior Registrar, Department of Paediatric Oncology

V. Ralph McCready, DSc, MRCP, FRCR
Consultant in Charge, Department of Nuclear Medicine

Ann C. Fullbrook, DCR (T), DRI
Radiographer, Department of Nuclear Medicine

The Royal Marsden Hospital, Downs Road, Sutton, Surrey SM2 5PT, UK

With contributions from
Sue L. Fielding, MSc
Senior Physicist, The Royal Marsden Hospital, Downs Road, Sutton, Surrey SM2 5PT, UK

Maggie A. Flower, MSc, PhD
Lecturer in Physics as Applied to Medicine, Institute of Cancer Research and The Royal Marsden
Hospital, Downs Road, Sutton, Surrey SM2 5PT, UK

B. G. Tyrwhitt-Drake, MA
Research and Development Manager, Pharmaceuticals Division, Amersham International plc,
Amersham Laboratories, White Lion Road, Amersham, Buckinghamshire HP7 9LL, UK

Cover illustration: Case 3, Stage IV Neuroblastoma, with isotope uptake seen in right lateral skull, posterior chest and abdomen, and posterior pelvis.

ISBN-13: 978-1-4471-1676-9   e-ISBN-13: 978-1-4471-1674-5
DOI: 10.1007/ 978-1-4471-1674-5

British Library Cataloguing in Publication Data
Moyes, Judy S. E., *1953–*
Neuroblastoma: mIBG in diagnosis and management
1. Children. Nervous system. Neuroblastomas I. Title II. McCready, V. R. (Victor Ralph) III. Fullbrook, Ann
C. 618.92'9948

Library of Congress Cataloging-in-Publication Data
Moyes, Judy S. E., *1953–*
Neuroblastoma: mIBG in diagnosis and management. Includes bibliographies and index.
1. Neuroblastoma—Radionuclide imaging. 2. Radiolabeled mIBG (Chemical)—Diagnostic use.
3. Neuroblastoma—Radiotherapy—Evaluation. 4. mIBG (Chemical)—Therapeutic use—Testing. I. McCready,
V. II. Fullbrook, Ann C. III. Title. [DNLM: 1. Idobenzen—diagnostic use. 2. Neuroblastoma—in infancy &
childhood. 3. Neuroblastoma—radionuclide imaging. QZ 380 M938n]
RC280.N4M69   1989   618.92'9948   88–33714

This work is subject to copyright. All rights are reserved, whether the whole or part of the material is concerned, specifically the rights of translation, reprinting, reuse of illustrations, recitation, broadcasting, reproduction on microfilms or in other ways, and storage in data banks. Duplication of this publication or parts thereof is only permitted under the provisions of the German Copyright Law of September 9, 1965, in its version of June 24, 1985, and a copyright fee must always be paid. Violations fall under the prosecution act of the German Copyright Law.

© Springer-Verlag Berlin Heidelberg 1989
Softcover reprint of the hardcover 1st edition 1989

The use of registered names, trademarks etc. in this publication does not imply, even in the absence of a specific statement, that such names are exempt from the relevant laws and regulations and therefore free for general use.

Product Liability: The publisher can give no guarantee for information about drug dosage and application thereof contained in this book. In every individual case the respective user must check its accuracy by consulting other pharmaceutical literature.

2128/3916–543210   Printed on acid-free paper

Preface

Neuroblastoma is the third most common malignancy of childhood, accounting for 8% of all cancers in patients under 15 years of age. In the majority of cases, by the time neuroblastoma is diagnosed, it has already spread from its site of origin to involve distant sites. Approximately 90% of cases of neuroblastoma can be diagnosed by a combination of techniques including detection of specific tumour markers in the urine, histopathological and immunocytological assessment of involved bone marrow and the 'characteristic' appearances of tumours demonstrated by computerised tomography and ultrasonography. However, despite this plethora of techniques, up to 10% of cases of neuroblastoma are still difficult to diagnose and rely on excisional biopsy of a site of disease. It was against this background that the scintigraphic localisation of neuroblastoma with the radiolabelled guanethidine analogue, mIBG, became available. With mIBG scintigraphy it is now possible to demonstrate the presence of neuroblastoma (and related tumours) at the primary site, soft tissue sites, in the bone marrow and in cortical bone, in a single investigation. The success of mIBG scintigraphy depends on many factors including the choice of isotope for labelling the mIBG, the equipment used to carry out the procedure, and the manipulation and interpretation of the information obtained.

At the Royal Marsden Hospital we have performed over 100 mIBG studies in children, and our advice has frequently been sought by other centres who are, or intend to become, actively engaged in this field. It was as a result of these enquiries that we decided to put together this book. We have not attempted to give a detailed dissertation and literature review of mIBG, but we have aimed to provide the basic information required when embarking on mIBG scintigraphy and a reference source of mIBG studies for comparison with normal and abnormal mIBG scintigrams.

Dr Judy Moyes is indebted to The Neuroblastoma Society for its financial support from October 1985 to October 1987, when she held the position of Neuroblastoma Society Research Fellow. We are grateful to Professor Timothy McElwain and Dr Simon Meller (both of The Royal Marsden Hospital) for allowing us to report on their patients. We would also like to thank Ms Sarah Chittenden (Physicist) for her constructive advice on Chapter 3, and Mrs Bernadette Cronin (Radiographer) for her help with the illustrations.

Finally thanks are due to Jamie Moyes without whose help, support and encouragement completion of the book would have been impossible. He gave up many weekends and evenings to care for our daughter Kate, in order that I could work on the book. For this we are all very grateful.

Sutton, 1988

Judy S. E. Moyes
V. Ralph McCready
Ann C. Fullbrook

Contents

Contents

Introduction

The idea that a radioactive isotope could be used to image or treat pathology arose in the 1940s when radioiodine and radioactive phosphorus became available to clinicians for the first time. The concept of a "magic bullet" was coined by Henry Wagner (Wagner 1975). It was envisaged that a series of radioactive magic bullets would be developed which could be used to diagnose and treat a whole series of diseases. The success of radioiodine therapy is well known but it is only after nearly 50 years that there are signs that this dream might become a reality.

The new developments encompass two areas – the development of antibodies to tumour-associated antigens (Larson 1985) and the use of meta-iodo-benzylguanidine (mIBG) for the diagnosis and treatment of neuroendocrine tumours. It has proved to be extremely difficult to develop agents which will concentrate in a particular tissue which can be labelled with a radionuclide. The obvious solution of labelling a precursor to a hormone or other substance produced by a tissue is generally impossible since most compounds in the body contain only the elements carbon, nitrogen, oxygen and hydrogen. Radioisotopes of these atoms all have a short half-life of 20 minutes or less, making synthesis of most compounds containing them impossible before most of the radioactivity has decayed away. An additional complication is that they are positron emitters which require a cyclotron for their production and a positron-emission tomography system for imaging, both of which for economic reasons are found only in large centres. The addition of a suitable radionuclide which emits a gamma ray with the correct energy for imaging or particle for therapy, generally alters the molecule sufficiently to change its chemical characteristics, making it no longer a precursor.

Biological techniques for localising and treating tumours have proved equally difficult to develop. So far an antigen specific to a particular tumour has not been found, although there are tumour-associated antigens to which antibodies can be prepared. In the case of neuroblastoma several centres have reported successful imaging with antibodies produced by immunising mice with human neural tissue or cultured human neuroblastoma (Horne et al. 1985; Cheung et al. 1987). Although the antibodies can be labelled with iodine-131, the low perfusion of tumours coupled with the lack of specificity results in a level of uptake which may give equivocal diagnostic results and a low chance of therapeutic success. Calculations suggest that it will always be difficult to achieve therapeutic uptakes of antibodies following intravenous administration (Vaughan et al. 1987) so it is particularly exciting that mIBG has been developed and applied to the diagnosis and treatment of neuroectodermal tumours. It is now the hope of nuclear medicine physicians that further similar compounds will follow.

For many years Beierwaltes and his group have studied methods of imaging the adrenal gland and its tumours (Beierwaltes et al. 1971). Attempts to use precursors of adrenaline as an imaging agent for adrenergic tumours showed that ^{14}C-dopamine and ^{14}C-labelled noradrenaline were the most likely to have sufficient uptake (Morales et al. 1976). It was some time before a radioiodine-labelled compound was ready for in-vivo use. Using a slightly

1

different approach, based on the functional similarity between the chromaffin cells of the adrenal medulla and the adrenergic neurons, Weiland and his colleagues in 1979 demonstrated good concentration of ^{131}I-ortho-iodobenzyldimethyl-2-hydroxyethyl ammonium in the dog adrenal gland. In the following year Weiland found a striking affinity for and retention in the dog adrenal medulla of ^{131}I-para-iodobenzylguanidine (Weiland et al. 1980). Subsequently this compound was used in the study of phaeochromocytoma (Valk et al. 1981). The high specificity (100%) and sensitivity (92.4%) (Shapiro et al. 1985) has confirmed the value of a lesion-specific radiopharmaceutical. A range of neuroendocrine tumours has been studied with mIBG, with varying degrees of sensitivity, including carcinoid (Hoefnagel 1987), non-secreting paragangliomas (Smit et al. 1984), medullary carcinoma of the thyroid (Endo et al. 1984), Sipple's syndrome (Perdrisot et al. 1988), chemodectomas, Merkel-cell skin cancer (Shapiro et al. 1986) and of course neuroblastoma, the subject of this book.

The use of mIBG in patients with neuroblastoma dates from 1983–84 when Kimmig at Heidelberg, and Feine at Tubingen, noticed that neuroblastomas actively absorbed and stored mIBG (Feine et al. 1987). A report of a multicentre study has shown that the sensitivity for primary neuroblastoma is over 90%, and for neuroblastoma with a high level of catecholamine excretion over 95%. The specificity is nearly 100%. Since then there have been many references to the use of mIBG for the diagnosis and therapy of neuroblastoma. Thus in a very short space of time another radiotherapeutic technique using an unsealed radiation source has become established. However, as yet experience is limited to very few centres and relatively few cases. Although in such a situation it is best to limit the numbers of centres performing diagnosis and therapy of these rare conditions on the grounds of economy and effectiveness, there is no doubt that mIBG imaging will spread throughout the world in the same way as did radioiodine therapy for differentiated carcinoma of the thyroid.

We have now performed over 100 mIBG studies (resulting in approximately 2000 images) in over 50 young children. After initial teething problems we feel we are able to consistently produce high quality images. As a result of our experience we have been frequently approached by other centres for advice on mIBG scintigraphy. The advice is usually related to two areas in particular. The first area is to assist those with no experience who are interested in setting up mIBG scintigraphy in their units. The second is to assist those units which are already performing mIBG examinations but are unhappy with the quality of images that are produced and have difficulty in assessing the variation in appearance of normal mIBG scintigrams. It is not our intention to convey that the techniques that we have outlined are the only ones that should be used; they are simply techniques that we have found to be successful and that other centres have also found success with.

The purpose of this book therefore is to present in a relatively small volume the background of the radiopharmaceutical mIBG and the disease neuroblastoma, the techniques for mIBG scanning, the normal and abnormal appearances of mIBG images, dosimetry calculations for mIBG, and an introduction to mIBG therapy for neuroblastoma.

References

Beierwaltes WH, Lieberman LM, Ansari AN (1971) Visualisation of the human adrenal glands by in vivo scintillation scanning. JAMA 216:275–277

Cheung N-KV, Neely JE, Landmeiar B, Nelson D, Miraldi F (1987) Targetting of ganglioside G_{D2} monoclonal antibody to neuroblastoma. J Nucl Med 28:1577–1583

Endo K, Shiomi K, Kasagi K et al. (1984) Imaging of medullary thyroid cancer with ^{131}I-mIBG. Lancet ii:233

Feine U, Muller-Schauenberg W, Treuner J et al. (1987) Meta-iodobenzylguanidine (mIBG) labelled with ^{123}I/^{131}I in neuroblastoma diagnosis and follow-up treatment with a review of diagnostic results of the International Workshop in Paediatric Oncology held in Rome, September 1986. Med Paediatr Oncol 15:181–187

Hoefnagel CA (1987) The role of ^{131}I-mIBG in the diagnosis and therapy of carcinoid. Eur J Nucl Med 13:187–191

Horne T, Granowski M, Dicks-Mireaux C et al. (1985) Neuroblastoma imaged with ^{123}I-meta-iodo-benzylguanidine and with ^{123}I-labelled monoclonal antibody UJ 13A against neural tissue. Br J Radiol 58:476–480

Larson SM (1985) Radiolabelled monoclonal anti-tumour antibodies in diagnosis and therapy. J Nucl Med 26:538–545

Morales JO, Beierwaltes WH, Counsell RE et al. (1976) The concentration of radioactivity from labelled epinephrine and its precursors in the dog adrenal medulla. J Nucl Med 8:800–809

Perdrisot R, Rohmer V, Lejeune JJ et al. (1988) Thyroid uptake of mIBG in Sipple's syndroma. Eur J Nucl Med 14:37–38

Shapiro B, Copp JE, Sisson JC et al. (1985) Iodine-131 meta-iodobenzylguanidine for the locating of suspected phaeo-chromocytoma: experience in 400 cases. J Nucl Med 26:576–585

Shapiro B, Von Moll L, McEwan A et al. (1986) I-131-meta-iodobenzylguanidine (MIBG) uptake by a wide range of neuro-endocrine tumors other than phaeochromocytoma and neuro-blastoma. J Nucl Med 27:908 (abstr)

Smit AJ, Van Essen LH, Hollenia H et al. (1984) ^{131}I-mIBG uptake in a non-secreting paraganglioma. J Nucl Med 25:984–986

Valk TW, Frager MS, Gross MD et al. (1981) Spectrum of phaeo-chromocytoma in multiple endocrine neoplasia: a scin-tigraphic portrayal using ^{131}I-metaiodobenzylguanidine. Ann Int Med 94:762–767

Vaughan ATM, Anderson P, Dykes PW et al. (1987) Limitations to the killing of tumours using radiolabelled antibodies. Br J Radiol 60:567–578

Wagner HJ (1975) Introduction. In: Wagner HJ (ed) Nuclear medicine. HP Publishing, New York, p XIII

Wieland DD, Swanson DP, Brown LE et al. (1979) Imaging the adrenal medulla with an I-131 labeled anti-adrenergic agent. J Nucl Med 20:155–158

Wieland DM, Wu J, Brown LE et al. (1980) Radiolabeled adren-ergic neuron-blocking agents: adrenomedullary imaging with [131I]iodobenzylguanidine. J Nucl Med 21:349–353

1 An Overview of Neuroblastoma

Neuroblastoma is a tumour of the sympathetic nervous system, originating from primitive neural crest cells that normally give rise to the adrenal medulla and sympathetic ganglia. It is the single most common, extracranial, solid, malignant tumour in children, with an incidence of 1–1.4 per 10 000 population.

Neuroblastoma is a tumour of young children, with approximately 50% being diagnosed before the age of 2 years, 80% by 5 years and 96% by 10 years of age (Bachmann 1972). It is not uncommonly diagnosed in the neonatal period, but rarely occurs in adulthood. Like many paediatric conditions, males are affected slightly more often than females with a male to female ratio of 1.2:1.

There has been no consistent association of neuroblastoma occurring with certain congenital defects (Miller 1968). Various cytogenetic abnormalities have been demonstrated in a number of children with neuroblastoma; however, no specific chromosomal pattern has been noted. There have been several reports of familial occurrence of neuroblastoma (Chatten and Voorhess 1967; Wagget et al. 1973; Gerson et al. 1974; Pegelow et al. 1975), and neuroblastoma has been described in children of parents with ganglioneuroma (Bond 1976).

Pathology

Neuroblastoma is unique in that it is more prone to spontaneous regression than any other human cancer. The neuroblast develops into three main cell types – the mature ganglion cell, the neuro-fibrous cell and the chromaffin cell – with many intermediate stages occurring in between. Tumours may be associated with each cell type, with the most common being the neuroblastoma, ganglioneuroma, neurofibroma and phaeochromocytoma. Neuroblastoma is the most primitive histologically. It is very cellular, composed of small round cells with scant cytoplasm which on light microscopy may be mistaken for other small round cell tumours, e.g. lymphoma, rhabdomyosarcoma and Ewing's sarcoma. Microscopically, the tumour varies from the profoundly primitive to one that is almost indistinguishable from normal neural tissue. The classical features of neuroblastoma are present in those tumours showing some evidence of maturation, and consist of rosette formation and neurofibrils. Neuroblastoma cells, unlike those of Ewing's tumour and rhabdomyosarcoma, rarely contain glycogen and therefore usually do not react with the glycogen stain, periodic acid-Schiff reagent (PAS).

Ganglioneuroma is composed of large, mature ganglion cells with abundant cytoplasm. Theoretically, intermediate within the spectrum of tumours, ranging from the benign ganglioneuroma to the malignant neuroblastoma, lies the ganglioneuroblastoma. However, ganglioneuroblastomas may show widely varying degrees of cellular maturation.

Light microscopy alone is frequently insufficient to make a firm diagnosis of neuroblastoma, and electron microscopy may be needed to illustrate the distinctive ultrastructure of the neuroblastoma cell and differentiate it from other small, round-cell tumours. The neuroblast has peripheral dendritic processes which contain longitudinally orientated microtubules. The cytoplasm contains small, spherical, membrane-bound granules with electron-dense cores. These granules contain catecholamines. A correlation has been shown between increased urinary excretion of catecholamines and the number of membrane-bound granules in the cytoplasm of the neuroblast (Misugi et al. 1968). Even the very poorly differentiated forms of neuroblastoma show the characteristic cytoplasmic structures of neurotubules and neurosecretory granules. It is into these granules that radiolabelled mIBG is concentrated, allowing the scintigraphic detection of sites of neuroblastoma.

Clinical Features

Neuroblastomas may arise in any anatomical site that is part of the sympathetic nervous system and this accounts for the wide variability in clinical signs and symptoms at diagnosis. In some children with widespread disease at presentation, it may be difficult to locate the exact site of origin of the tumour. In approximately 70% of cases the primary site is in the retroperitoneal region, arising from the adrenal medulla or sympathetic ganglia (cervical, thoracic or pelvic) (Voûte et al. 1987).

The primary tumour is most frequently in the abdomen, and therefore abdominal distension or an abdominal mass commonly occurs, and may be associated with nausea, vomiting, abdominal pain, localised tenderness, urinary retention or a disturbance of bowel habit. Pelvic tumours may be palpable on rectal examination, and may also produce urinary symptoms as well as a change in bowel habit.

Tumours arising in the posterior mediastinum can give rise to dysphagia, respiratory distress and chest infections. Alternatively, they may be asymptomatic and noted on a chest radiograph performed for other reasons.

Cervical lymphadenopathy may be a primary site or a metastatic site of disease. Usually it is noted as an asymptomatic swelling; however, it may produce an ipsilateral Horner's syndrome (which has also been noted with mediastinal lymph-node enlargement).

Neuroblastoma arising from a paravertebral sympathetic ganglion has a tendency to grow through the intervertebral foramina to form an intraspinal component, resulting in what is commonly known as a "dumb-bell" tumour. These tumours frequently have neurological sequelae. Early symptoms include hypotonia, muscle atrophy, areflexia, hyper-reflexia and spasticity. Later, cord compression may occur, with paralysis, weakness of an extremity and incontinence. The latter situation requires emergency treatment to prevent permanent damage. However, in approximately 40% of cases the intraspinal component is not clinically apparent (Akwari et al. 1978).

Rarely, the presenting features may be those of unilateral nasal obstruction and epistaxis due to the primary tumour originating in the olfactory bulb. This is known as an aesthesioneuroblastoma. It rarely presents in childhood, and has a peak incidence in the second decade of life.

Metastatic skin lesions may be common presenting findings in the neonatal period. The subcutaneous bluish nodules, sometimes known as "blueberry muffins", are erythematous for two to three minutes after palpation and then blanch, presumably secondary to vasoconstriction due to release of catecholamines from the tumour cells.

The common sites for metastatic disease in patients other than neonates include the liver, bone and bone marrow. Often the first signs of illness are symptoms referable to skeletal involvement, with bone pain being particularly prevalent. More than 50% of children at diagnosis will have bone marrow involvement. This may present as pallor, increased susceptibility to infections and a tendency to bruise, resulting from anaemia, neutropenia and thrombocytopenia, respectively. Metastatic retrobulbar soft-tissue involvement results in periorbital oedema and proptosis, with periorbital bruising, producing the "raccoon facies" which is not uncommonly seen.

An uncommon, but well-described, association is that of acute myoclonic encephalopathy with neuroblastoma. The symptoms of opsoclonus (rapid multidirectional eye movements), myoclonus, and truncal ataxia in the absence of raised intracranial pressure, may precede the development of clinical neuroblastoma by some years in some patients.

Finally, some symptoms of neuroblastoma result from its metabolic activity. Hypertension, flushing, periods of excessive sweating, and irritability are caused by excessive production and excretion of catecholamines. Persistent, intractable, watery diarrhoea may occur as a result of the tumour's excretion of the enterohormone, vasoactive intestinal peptide.

Despite this plethora of possible clinical signs and symptoms, the commonest presentation of all is the child who is non-specifically unwell with fevers, anorexia, weight loss, pallor and irritability.

Diagnostic Features

Haematology and Biochemistry

1. Anaemia, neutropenia and thrombocytopenia may be present as a result of infiltration of the bone marrow by neuroblastoma.

2. The catecholamines dopamine, noradrenaline and adrenaline play an important role in the function of the sympathetic nervous system, and as has already been described they are present in the neurosecretory granules of the cytoplasm of the neuroblast. Therefore it is not surprising that more than 90% of children with neuroblastoma produce excessive amounts of these catecholamines and/or their metabolites. The metabolites include dihydroxyphenylalanine (DOPA), normetanephrine, 3-methoxytyramine, homovanilic acid (HVA), and vanillylmandelic acid (VMA). These substances are excreted in the urine, and therefore their levels can be measured and thus serve as tumour markers. However, it should be noted that some children (approximately 5%) do not excrete increased levels of catecholamines. The percentage of children who are quoted as being non-excretors varies between different studies; the discrepancy between the studies is due in part to the fact that different authors measure limited numbers of DOPA metabolites. The more metabolites that are measured the more likely that the patient is found to be excreting raised levels of some metabolite.

3. Raised levels of neuron-specific enolase (NSE) in the serum are found at diagnosis, and the level has been shown to correlate with the stage of the disease at diagnosis (Zeltzer et al. 1985).

4. The serum ferritin has also been found to be raised at diagnosis in some patients. The degree of increase appears to correlate with the prognosis in individual patients.

Histopathology

The histopathology of neuroblastoma has already been discussed in some detail. To assess possible bone marrow infiltration by neuroblastoma, aspirations and trephines from the posterior iliac crests should be performed. The appearances are not dissimilar from leukaemia or Ewing's sarcoma, but the neuroblastoma cells are more likely to occur in clumps or rosettes.

Radiological Studies

The location of the primary site will determine the particular studies to be performed. Usually a plain radiograph of the chest or abdomen is indicated. In all patients a ^{99m}Tc-MDP bone scan should be performed to assess bony involvement, and in some institutions a skeletal survey may be undertaken as well. A computed tomographic (CT) scan of the area of the primary site is indicated. In those patients with a tumour that lies close to the vertebral column, a CT myelogram will also be necessary to exclude the possibility of intraspinal extension of the tumour. Ultrasound of the primary site is also usually undertaken, and any calcification within the tumour should be noted (as this commonly occurs with neuroblastoma).

Despite this plethora of investigations which are available to diagnose and stage neuroblastoma, for some cases diagnosis still remains difficult. Therefore, when the radiolabelled guanethidine analogue, ^{131}I-mIBG, was shown to be concentrated by neuroblastoma, it quickly became established as a specific and sensitive method of detecting the disease. For this reason mIBG scintigraphy has become part of the initial routine investigations in the detection of residual, recurrent or metastatic disease.

Clinical Staging

Two main staging systems have been used for neuroblastoma, the TNM system (International Union against Cancer 1985) and staging according to Evans et al. (1971). In the case studies described in this book the Evans system has been used, and therefore only this system will be described.

Stage I	Tumour confined to the organ or structure of origin.
Stage II	Tumour with regional spread that does not cross the midline; ipsilateral lymph nodes may be involved.
Stage III	Regional tumour crossing the midline; bilateral lymph nodes may be involved.
Stage IV	Tumour with metastases to distant discontiguous sites such as lymph nodes, bone and bone marrow, organs and soft tissue.
Stage IVs	Localised primary tumour and disseminated disease limited to liver, skin and bone marrow.

The staging of neuroblastoma is important since it provides information regarding prognosis. It is also useful not only as a basis for the selection of treatment, but in the evaluation of treatment as well.

Prognostic Features

There are several factors which are taken into account, when assessing the prognosis in individual patients with neuroblastoma. The stage of the disease at diagnosis is the most important factor, with stage III and IV disease having a much worse prognosis than stage I or II, and stage IVs disease having an excellent prognosis.

The age of the patient at diagnosis is inversely related to survival, with children under 1 year of age at diagnosis having a better outcome irrespective of their stage at diagnosis.

The site of the primary tumour also affects the outcome. The outlook is worse for tumours which arise in the adrenal gland than for those in which the primary site is in the cervical, thoracic or pelvic sympathetic chains.

Other prognostic factors include the pattern of excretion of catecholamines, and the levels of neuron-specific enolase and ferritin at diagnosis.

Treatment

Different treatment programmes are needed for different stages of the disease. However, it is not the purpose of this chapter to enter into a detailed discussion on the treatment protocols currently available, and the survival rates associated with each protocol.

For stage I and II disease complete excision is usually all that is required, followed by careful monitoring of the patient to ensure that relapse does not occur.

For stage III and IV disease, which encompasses the majority of patients, the approach that is commonly employed involves three stages. The initial step is treatment with multi-agent chemotherapy. This is followed by surgical excision of the primary site, and in some institutions external beam radiotherapy. The final stage is treatment with high-dose chemotherapy followed by autologous bone marrow rescue. For the initial chemotherapy many different protocols are available, but the one which has gained acceptance and been successfully used

throughout Europe is the OPEC regimen (Appendix A) which involves the use of four agents – vincristine, cyclophosphamide, etoposide and cisplatin. These are given in combination for six to ten courses usually, with an interval of approximately three weeks between courses. After this initial chemotherapy, if excision (partial or total) is thought to be possible, it should be aggressive with removal of as much of the tumour as possible. The high-dose chemotherapy programmes available are varied. At The Royal Marsden Hospital we use high-dose melphalan (Appendix B) which was pioneered by McElwain et al. (1979). The bone marrow rescue is performed with the patients own marrow, which may or may not have been "cleaned" before re-infusion, to remove any neuroblastoma cells present. Various forms of cleaning exist, including cell-separation methods (Figdor et al. 1981), and the use of magnetic beads coupled to monoclonal antibodies directed against neuroblastoma cells (Kemshead et al. 1984).

Despite these intensive treatment programmes the survival for stage IV neuroblastoma remains poor, with three-year survival being only approximately 30%–40%. Therefore, when the use of radio-labelled mIBG was shown to be a specific and sensitive method of detecting neuroblastoma, the possibility that it might also be used as a form of targetted radiotherapy for this disease was greeted with great enthusiasm.

References

Akwari OE, Payne WS, Onofrio BM et al. (1978) Dumbbell neurogenic tumours of the mediastinum. Diagnosis and management. Mayo Clin Proc 53:353–358

Bachmann KD (1972) Tumoren des sympathischen Nervensystems. In: Schmid F (ed) Tumoren im Kindesalter. Springer, Berlin Heidelberg New York, p328 (Handbuch der Kinderheilkunde, vol 8/2)

Bond JV (1976) Familial neuroblastoma and ganglioneuroma. JAMA 236:561–562

Chatten J, Voorhess ML (1967) Familial neuroblastoma: report of a kindred with multiple disorders, including neuroblastoma in four siblings. N Engl J Med 227:1230–1236

Evans AE, D'Angio GJ, Randolph J (1971) A proposed staging for children with neuroblastoma: Children's Cancer Study Group A. Cancer 27:374–378

Figdor CG, Bont WS, de Vries JE et al. (1981) Isolation of large numbers of highly purified lymphocytes and monocytes with a modified centrifugal elutriation technique. J Immunol Methods 40:275–288

Gerson JM, Chatten J, Eisman S (1974) Familial neuroblastoma – a follow-up. N Engl J Med 290:1487

References

International Union against Cancer (UICC) (1985) TNM-atlas, illustrated guide to the TNM/pTNM-classification of malignant tumours. 2nd ed. UICC, Geneva

Kemshead JT, Treleavan JG, Gibson FM et al. (1984) Removal of neuroblastoma cells from bone marrow with monoclonal antibodies conjugated to magnetic microspheres. Lancet 1:70–73

McElwain TJ, Hedley DW, Gordon MY et al. (1979) High-dose melphalan and non-cryopreserved autologous bone marrow treatment of malignant melanoma and neuroblastoma. Exp Haematol 7 (Suppl 5):360

Miller RW (1968) Relation between cancer and congenital defects: an epidemiological evaluation. J Natl Cancer Inst 40:1079–1085

Misugi K, Misugi N, Newton WA (1968) Fine ultrastructural study of neuroblastoma, ganglioneuroblastoma, and phaeochromocytoma. Arch Pathol (Chicago) 86:160–170

Pegelow CH, Ebbin AJ, Powars D et al. (1975) Familial neuroblastoma. J Pediatr 87:763–765

Voûte PA, de Kraker J, Burgers JMV (1987) Tumours of the sympathetic nervous system – neuroblastoma, ganglioneuroma and phaeochromocytoma. In: Voûte PA, Barrett A, Bloom HJG, Lemerle J, Neidhardt MK (eds) Cancer in children – clinical management. Springer, Berlin Heidelberg New York Tokyo, pp 238–251

Wagget J, Aherne G, Aherne W (1973) Familial neuroblastoma: report of two sib pairs. Arch Dis Child 48:63–66

Zelter PM, Marangos PJ, Sather H et al. (1985) Prognostic importance of serum neuron specific enolase in local and widespread neuroblastoma. Prog Clin Biol Res 175:319–329

2 Chemistry and Pharmacy of mIBG

B. G. Tyrwhitt-Drake

Pharmacology

As early as 1967 attempts were made to develop radiopharmaceuticals for imaging the adrenal medulla, based upon the properties of that tissue to synthesize, store and secrete catecholamines. One approach has been to develop analogues of the hypotensive drug guanethidine, which is known to act by depletion of noradrenaline from storage granules as well as interfering with the normal catecholamine release mechanism in response to an evoked potential (Maxwell and Wastila 1977). Studies of ^{14}C-guanethidine uptake in dogs showed that this compound has a high affinity for the adrenal medulla; however, there are no straightforward methods for radiolabelling guanethidine with a suitable gamma-emitting isotope. Attention therefore focused on the development of guanethidine analogues which exhibited similar biodistribution but which could be labelled for routine imaging in a nuclear medicine department.

In 1980 Wieland et al. developed the iodobenzylguanidine series which have structural similarities to both guanethidine and the endogenous catecholamines (Fig. 2.1). Furthermore, these compounds could be radiolabelled with either ^{123}I or ^{131}I, allowing their biodistribution in animals and man to be imaged with the gamma camera. The meta-iodobenzylguanidine (mIBG) isomer was shown to have advantages over the para-iodobenzylguanidine isomer in imaging studies

(Wieland et al. 1981), probably due to its greater resistance to in-vivo de-iodination, and it is mIBG which has been subsequently widely studied and accepted as an imaging agent for normal and pathological catecholamine concentrations in man.

For many of the storage, release and uptake mechanisms of endogenous catecholamines, mIBG is known to be a marker. When noradrenaline is released from storage granules in response to an action potential (Fig. 2.2) some is taken up by an active process, Uptake 1, into the cytoplasmic pool from where it can be re-assembled into storage granules. The mIBG is probably taken up by the same process as noradrenaline (Jaques et al. 1984, 1987) and similarly stored and released from granules (Wieland et al. 1981; Jaques and Tobes 1985; Gagnier et al. 1986).

The clinical applications for radiolabelled mIBG therefore relate to its ability to image functional normalities and abnormalities of the catecholamine pool. Tissues rich in sympathetic nerves, such as the myocardium have been successfully imaged with ^{123}I-mIBG (Sisson et al. 1987), and the characteristic uptake and retention of mIBG in adrenal tissues has been shown to hold true for a human neuroblastoma cell line (Buck et al. 1985). Figure 2.2 illustrates the uptake, synthesis, storage and release of noradrenaline at an adrenergic nerve terminal, ignoring catabolic enzymes.

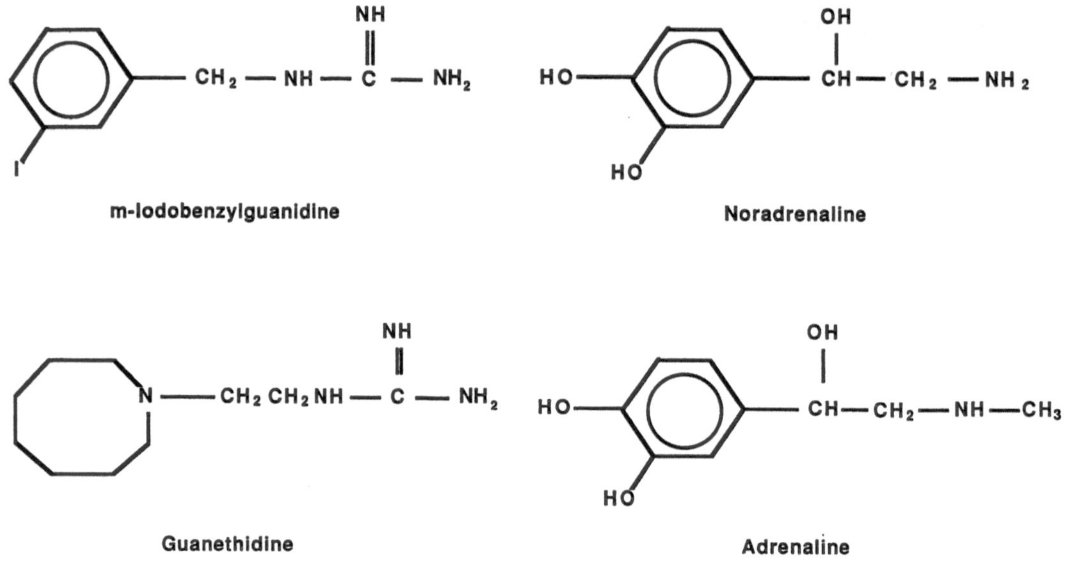

Fig. 2.1. Guanethidine shows a high affinity for the dog adrenal medulla but cannot be labelled with a gamma-emitting radioisotope. mIBG is an analogue of guanethidine with an iodine atom which can be substituted with radioiodine. The chemical formulae of adrenaline and its precursor noradrenaline are shown on the right.

Radiolabelled mIBG Products

When mIBG is radiolabelled with a suitable isotope of iodine, it can be expected to accumulate in normal tissues rich in sympathetic nerve tissue and in tumours with high catecholamine levels. The choice of iodine isotope is in practice limited to either ^{123}I or ^{131}I for imaging, and to ^{131}I for therapeutic irradiation of tumours (Table 2.1).

The physical properties of ^{123}I-mIBG make it the radiopharmaceutical of choice for imaging purposes. However, its advantages in terms of emissions and lower radiation doses are offset by higher costs and poorer availability. [123]I is cyclotron-produced, which accounts for its relatively high price, and care needs to be exercised, from a dosimetry point of view, that the level of [124]I and ^{125}I contamination is acceptable.

Table 2.1. Characteristics of radioiodine labels used in mIBG studies

Isotope	Half-life	Type of decay	Particle energies and transition		Electromagnetic transitions	
			Energy (MeV)	Transition probability (%)	Photon energy (MeV)	Photons emitted (%)
[131]I	8.04 days	β-	0.247	1.8	0.080	2.4
			0.304	0.6	0.284	5.9
			0.334	7.2	0.364	81.8
			0.606	98.7	0.637	7.2
			0.806	0.7	0.723	1.8
[123]I	13.2 hours	Electron capture		100	0.0272 0.0274 0.031 }	86
					0.159	83.4
					0.529	1.4

12

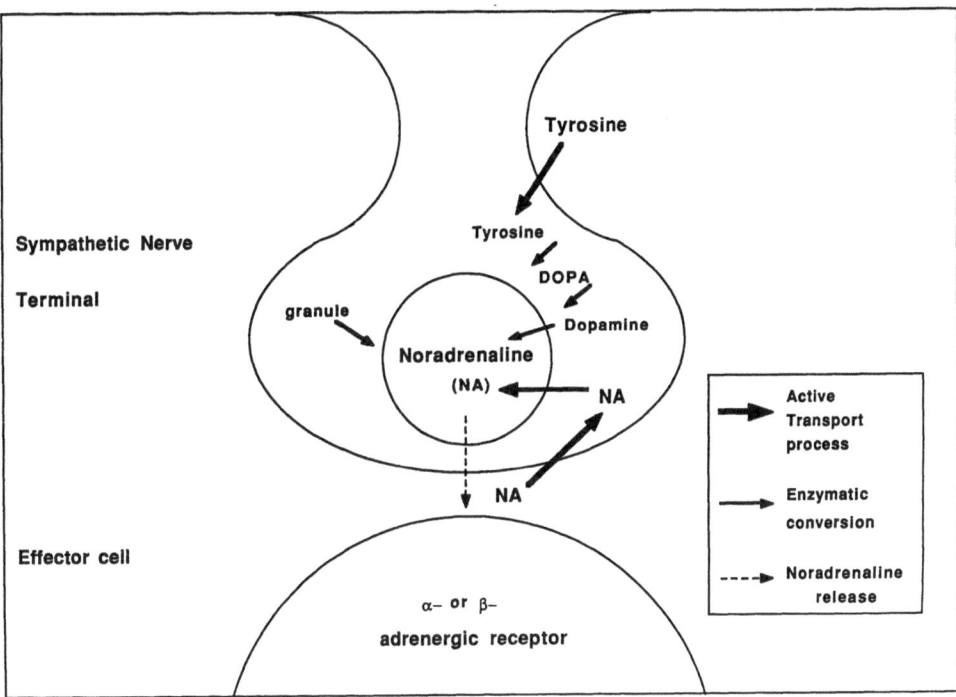

Fig. 2.2. Diagrammatic representation of the catecholamine pathways.

Formulations and Stability of mIBG

Both ^{123}I-mIBG and ^{131}I-mIBG are normally formulated as sterile aqueous solutions in isotonic saline for injection. The solutions may contain 10 mg/ml of benzyl alcohol as a stabiliser to retard radiation decomposition in the vial. The major radiochemical impurity in ^{123}I-mIBG and ^{131}I-mIBG is free iodide, formed by radiolysis. Provided that the radioactive concentration of ^{131}I-mIBG solutions is less than 18 MBq/ml (0.5 mCi/ml) at reference and the specific activity is less than 185 MBq/mg (5 mCi/mg) at reference, levels of free iodide of ^{131}I should stay below 5% up to the expiry date for the product when stored at room temperature. Similar limits for ^{123}I-mIBG of less than 2 mCi/mg at reference for specific activity have been found (Amersham International, unpublished data). However, since it is known that radioactive mIBG solutions decompose more rapidly at elevated temperatures and in strong light, solutions should normally be stored at 2–8 °C in the dark.

Therapeutic doses of ^{131}I-mIBG are formulated at higher specific activities and radioactive concentrations. Typical values at reference dates are 10 mCi/ml for radioactive concentration and 1.1 GBq/mg (30 mCi/mg) for specific activity. These products are normally shipped in dry ice to prevent free iodide formation during transport and storage. Figure 2.3 shows the rapid formation of free iodide in a batch of therapeutic ^{131}I-mIBG stored at both room temperature and in dry ice.

Therapeutic ^{131}I-mIBG doses should be thawed by placing them in a water bath held below 50 °C for 1 hour, then diluted into 50 ml of 0.9% sterile sodium chloride for injection. Therapy doses are generally delivered to the patient in less than two hours to avoid excessive radiolytic decomposition of the diluted ^{131}I-mIBG in the infusion set.

The measurement of the radiochemical purity of ^{123}I-mIBG and ^{131}I-mIBG solutions by thin-layer chromatography is notoriously difficult and results may be very inaccurate. If measurement of radiochemical purity is to be made prior to administration, a suitable high-performance liquid chromatographic or electrophoresis system should be used (Maxwell and Wastila 1977).

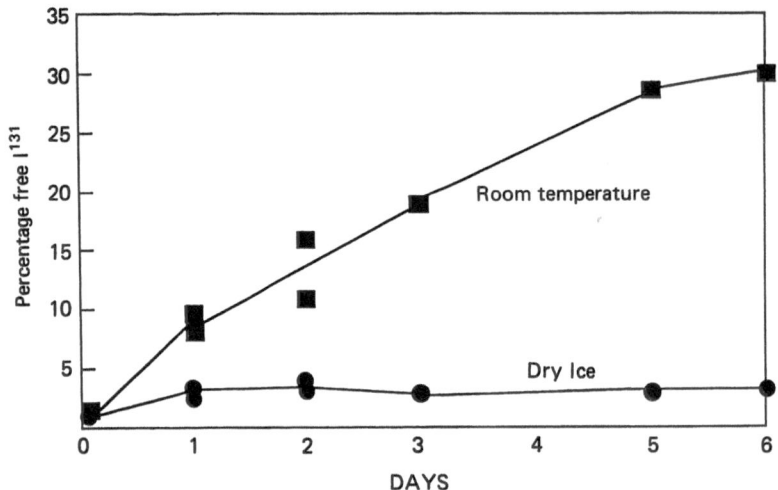

Fig. 2.3. Release of free iodine from ^{131}I-mIBG at room temperature and when stored in dry ice.

Toxicology

Acute toxicology studies with non-radioactive mIBG formulations in rats have shown no mortalities at 1200 times the normal human dose which contains 1 mg of mIBG (Amersham International, unpublished data). At a dose of 1 mg in man it is unlikely that the classical pharmacological effects of mIBG will be seen.

Conclusion

There are few compounds which can be labelled with a suitable gamma- or beta-emitting radionuclide which can be used to trace a human metabolic pathway, and mIBG is one of the first to trace a specific biochemical process. It is fortunate that it can be easily labelled with radioisotopes of iodine which are suitable for imaging (^{123}I), therapy (^{131}I), and positron emission tomography (^{124}I). The paucity of compounds available for tracing other metabolic processes is a reflection of the chemical difficulty in incorporating a suitable gamma- or beta-emitting radiolabel into the molecule – one that has no effect on the essential biochemical properties. This is in contrast to compounds where one can replace an atom of carbon, nitrogen or oxygen with a positron emitting radionuclide. However, since access to the necessary cyclotron is limited to only a few selected centres, the recent introduction of mIBG is welcome.

References

Buck J, Bruchelt G, Girgert R, et al. (1985) Specific uptake of m-[^{125}I] iodobenzylguanidine in the human neuroblastoma cell line SK-N-SH. Cancer Res 85:6366-6370

Gagnier B, Rosin MP, Scherman D, et al. (1986) Uptake of meta-iodobenzylguanidine by bovine chromaffin granule membranes. Molec Pharmacol 29:275-280

Jaques S, Tobes MC (1985) Comparison of the secretory mechanisms of meta-iodobenzylguanidine (mIBG) and norepinephrine (NE) from cultured bovine adrenomedullary cells. J Nucl Med 26:17

Jaques S. Tobes MC, Sisson JC (1984) Comparison of the sodium dependency of uptake of meta-iodobenzylguanidine and norepinephrine into cultured bovine adrenomedullary cells. Molec Pharmacol 26:539–546

Jaques S, Tobes MC, Sisson JC (1987) Sodium dependency of uptake of norepinephrine and m-iodobenzylguanidine into cultured human pheochromocytoma cells: evidence for uptake-one. Cancer Res 47:3920–3928

Maxwell RA, Wastila WB (1977) Acute hypertensive agents. In Gross F (ed) Handbook of experimental pharmacology, Springer, Berlin, Heidelberg, New York, vol 39. p 161

Sisson JC, Shapiro B. Meyers L et al. (1987) Meta-iodobenzylguanidine to map scintigraphically the adrenergic nervous system in man. J Nucl Med 28:10

Wieland DM, Wu J-L, Brown LE et al. (1980) Radiolabeled adrenergic neuron-blocking agents: adrenomedullary imaging with [^{131}I]iodobenzylguanidine. J Nucl Med 21:349–353

Wieland DM, Brown LE, Tobes MC et al. (1981) Imaging the primate adrenal medullae with [^{123}I] and [^{131}I]meta-iodobenzylguanidine: concise communication. J Nucl Med 22:358–364

3 Techniques for Imaging with mIBG

Imaging with mIBG has the advantage that the abnormality is seen as an area of increased radioactivity in a background of less activity, facilitating detection and interpretation. The mIBG images have been shown, by many centres, to demonstrate lesions not visible on other modalities; therefore mIBG scintigraphy is now accepted by most paediatric oncologists as potentially a very valuable additional technique for accurate staging of neuroblastoma, provided high-quality images are produced. Special imaging techniques and optimal conditions are required to reduce the number of poor-quality images as these give equivocal results.

However, mIBG scintigraphy has a second, equally important role to play in the disease neuroblastoma. It forms the basis on which decisions will be made regarding targetted radiotherapy with mIBG.

Patient Preparation

Imaging with mIBG is performed in the entire paediatric age group, but is more commonly performed on young children (under the age of 4 years) since neuroblastoma occurs more frequently in infants and toddlers. It is crucial that the patient lies completely motionless for the period of the examination. It is important therefore to explain what will happen during the test, to allay any apprehension produced by precautions necessary when dealing with radioactivity, and to help keep the patient relaxed and still during the examination. The presence of parents is valuable to give moral support and company, and to provide light entertainment if necessary (e.g. reading to the child) to relieve boredom. This will prevent fidgeting which is liable to occur during what has to be a lengthy procedure.

Sedation

For infants or babies sedation is usually advised. We use an oral "cocktail" (Appendix C) which has been prepared by our pharmacy and has been found to provide good sedation, allowing repositioning of the child by the radiographer which is necessary to obtain good images of the entire body, whilst allowing the child to "wake up" within a few hours of the procedure and return home if appropriate.

Thyroid Blockade

To prevent uptake of radioiodine into the thyroid gland as a result of in-vivo de-iodination of the radiolabelled mIBG, the thyroid should be blocked by prior administration of appropriate medication. We commonly use Lugol's iodine, 0.2 ml by mouth three times a day (or 0.6 ml as a once daily dose), starting 24–48 hours before administration of the radiopharmaceutical and continuing for 5 days if the ^{123}I isotope, and 7 days if the ^{131}I isotope, is being used. Appendix D gives further details regarding other suitable preparations which may be used instead of Lugol's iodine.

15

Medicines which Interfere with Uptake of mIBG

The mechanism by which mIBG is taken up by sympatho-adrenal tissue has already been described in Chapter 2. There are many drugs/compounds which on a theoretical basis could interfere with the concentration of mIBG by neuroblastoma, for example by interfering with the uptake mechanisms or acting as competitive inhibitors. It has now been shown that the simultaneous administration of some medicines inhibits the uptake of mIBG, resulting in false-negative mIBG studies. Therefore the discontinuation of these medicines 2–6 weeks before administration of the radiopharmaceutical should be considered if this is clinically possible. The classes of drugs which have interfered with the uptake of mIBG are the tricyclic antidepressants and related drugs, some antihypertensives, phenothiazines, amphetamines and particularly some nasal decongestants and cough preparations which can be bought without a prescription. A full list of medications which we advise our patients to avoid for a minimum of two weeks before mIBG scintigraphy is given in Appendix E.

Radiopharmaceuticals

For imaging purposes, mIBG may be radiolabelled with either ^{123}I or ^{131}I. The ^{131}I-mIBG comes as a sterile aqueous solution containing 5 mg/ml of sodium chloride and 10 mg/ml of benzyl alcohol. The pH of the solution lies within the range 4.0–7.0. The ^{123}I-mIBG similarly is formulated in isotonic saline with each millilitre containing less than 4 mg of mIBG. In the Amersham International product the free iodine at expiry is not more than 5%.

Choice of Radionuclide

The quality of any radionuclide image depends upon the total number of photons collected and the scattering characteristics of the radionuclide in the body.

There are a number of advantages of ^{123}I over ^{131}I as a radiolabel for mIBG. The energy of the principal gamma ray emitted by ^{123}I is 159 keV, whilst that of ^{131}I is much higher at 364 keV. Most modern gamma cameras are constructed in such a way as to optimise their performance (e.g. sensitivity, uniformity and resolution) for use with ^{99m}Tc, which has its photopeak at 140 keV. Since the photopeak energy of ^{123}I is very close to this value, the gamma cameras are effectively optimised for use with ^{123}I also. However, their performance is very much poorer at higher energies such as that of ^{131}I. In particular, the thickness of the sodium iodide crystal in a gamma camera optimised for ^{99m}Tc imaging, may be of the order of a quarter of an inch. This is too thin to efficiently image high-energy gamma rays, such as those from ^{131}I, since most of them will pass straight through the crystal without interacting. Furthermore, imaging of the 364 keV of ^{131}I requires the use of a high-energy collimator which has thick lead septa to prevent penetration of scattered radiation. The sensitivity of such collimators is poor, which adds to the problem of low counting efficiency previously described. However, imaging of ^{123}I gamma rays may be performed with a low-energy, high-resolution collimator with thin septa (such as may be used for ^{99m}Tc), resulting in both greater sensitivity and resolution.

In addition, with ^{123}I twenty times as much activity may be administered to the patient compared with ^{131}I for the same absorbed radiation dose: 370 MBq (10 mCi) of ^{123}I-mIBG delivers approximately the same radiation absorbed dose as 18 MBq (0.5 mCi) of ^{131}I-mIBG. This results in a higher photon flux reaching the gamma camera when ^{123}I is used. These and other factors all contribute to those images obtained using ^{123}I containing more counts, and having better uniformity and resolution than those obtained using ^{131}I. Higher count densities are a great advantage when performing single-photon emission computed tomography (SPECT), so ^{123}I is particularly to be preferred to ^{131}I for SPECT studies.

Thus we feel that ^{123}I-mIBG is the radiopharmaceutical of choice when performing mIBG scintigraphy as an investigation for diagnosis, staging or routine follow-up of children with neuroblastoma, or when SPECT is being performed. However, since some centres are unable to obtain ^{123}I-mIBG, ^{131}I-mIBG has to be used and it is fair to say that this radiopharmaceutical will also give images which can provide necessary information for diagnosis and follow-up.

^{131}I-mIBG is essential, however, for scans being performed for dosimetry estimation purposes prior to targetted radiotherapy with ^{131}I-mIBG.

Activity of Radiopharmaceutical

The total activity that can be administered is limited by the permissible radiation dose. In the United Kingdom the usual activity permitted when using ^{131}I-mIBG is 18.55–37.0 MBq (0.5–1.0 mCi) and when using ^{123}I-mIBG up to 370 MBq (10 mCi). In our patients we follow the guidelines shown in Table 3.1.

Table 3.1. Activity of radiopharmaceutical to be administered

Radiopharma-ceutical	Patient weight	Activity to be administered
^{123}I-mIBG	< 10 kg	75 MBq (2 mCi)
^{123}I-mIBG	> 10 kg	185 MBq (5 mCi)
^{131}I-mIBG	any weight	18 MBq (0.5 mCi)

Gamma Camera Technique

Since the information density varies throughout the body and from patient to patient following administration of mIBG, it is essential to perform imaging with a computer-based gamma camera. This enables the data acquired to be stored and subsequently viewed using the optimum display settings. For example, the upper and lower window levels may be altered to demonstrate small changes in uptake in areas of both increased radioactivity (hot) and decreased radioactivity (cold). Most of the images reproduced in this book were acquired using the International General Electric Starcam system – a modern, digital gamma camera and computer system combined.

Collimator

A low-energy, high-resolution, parallel-hole collimator is used when imaging with ^{123}I-mIBG. For imaging with ^{131}I-mIBG a high-energy, parallel-hole collimator is used.

Quality Control

To achieve the best results possible when imaging it is essential that the gamma camera is performing optimally. This is ensured by regular quality control.

Daily qualitative checks of uniformity are carried out using a ^{57}Co flood source to acquire images of 1 000 000 counts on a 128×128 matrix. Weekly qualitative checks of resolution and linearity are carried out using the ^{57}Co flood source and a lead bar phantom with minimum bar size and spacing of 2 mm. These images are also acquired for 1 000 000 counts, but with a matrix size of 256×256. Regular quantitative checks of intrinsic uniformity are performed using both ^{99m}Tc and ^{131}I point sources.

Flood data are acquired to a total of 30 000 000 counts on a 64×64 matrix, and are analysed according to the method laid down by the National Electrical Manufacturers Association (NEMA). Typically the values of non-uniformity obtained on our Starcam system are less than $\pm 3\%$ for the central field of view, and less than $\pm 8\%$ for the useful fields of view of the cameras. In addition to the above, occasional checks are made to ensure that the system sensitivity and the intrinsic resolution and linearity of the camera agree with the manufacturer's specifications and do not vary substantially with time.

For tomographic imaging the position of the centre of rotation of the camera must also be regularly checked and should not vary substantially. This is done by imaging a small point source placed at the approximate centre of rotation. A tomographic acquisition is performed consisting of 32 views over 360° on a 64×64 matrix with 20 000–30 000 counts in each view. System software is used to calculate the centre of rotation. It is also important to correct tomographic images for any non-uniformity (e.g. due to collimators or crystal sensitivity) which can produce ring artefacts in the reconstructed images. This is done by acquiring a flood field image using the same radioisotope and collimator that is used for the patient's mIBG study. A flood image of 30 000 000 counts is acquired on a 128×128 matrix, and system software is provided to use the image to correct the tomographic scan appropriately. It should be noted that it is possible to use ^{99m}Tc flood images to correct the ^{123}I tomographic images, since the gamma-camera response to the two isotopes is very similar.

Energy Windows

The choice of energy window width and centring is an important consideration. A narrow energy window improves the resolution of the image by rejecting scattered photons, but decreases the sensitivity (the number of counts which can be acquired during the imaging procedure). An image which has fewer counts but includes less scatter is probably better than the reverse. To achieve this some departments have therefore suggested the use of asymmetric energy windows which are centred above the photopeak. On the Starcam system we use a 20% width energy window centred directly on the photopeak for imaging with ^{123}I. For ^{131}I, however, we use a 12% width window, offset by 1% to the high-energy side of the 364 keV photopeak (where percentages are expressed relative to the photopeak value). We have found these energy windows produce the optimum images provided the appropriate energy corrections are used during the acquisition.

Energy corrections may be derived for any isotope using system software and are performed monthly as part of our quality control procedure. For imaging with ^{131}I, a ^{131}I energy correction is used; but for ^{123}I imaging we have found that it is adequate to use an energy correction derived for ^{99m}Tc.

Administration of mIBG

Radiolabelled mIBG is a noradrenaline analogue and therefore the theoretical possibility exists that the mIBG may displace noradrenaline from the storage granules, resulting in a surge in noradrenaline levels and possibly precipitating a hypertensive crisis. This is more likely to occur with phaeochromocytoma than neuroblastoma; however, it is advised that administration should be by slow intravenous injection over at least 30 seconds. In the small, wriggling child this may be difficult, and therefore to avoid extravasation of the radiopharmaceutical during administration, we restrain the child by wrapping in a sheet and have extra personnel available to assist for this brief period, if necessary.

Planar Imaging

Whole-body imaging is required for the full assessment of patients with neuroblastoma. A series of overlapping planer views can be taken using either preset fixed imaging times or preset counts. With the high count rates obtained with ^{123}I, images with the required information density can be obtained in a few minutes; however, the low count rate resulting from ^{131}I means that it may take as long as 20 minutes to obtain satisfactory images, and considerably longer for views of certain areas, for example the lower limbs. We have adopted a policy of acquiring each image for 10 minutes when we are using the ^{123}I isotope, and 20 minutes for the ^{131}I isotope, to get the best information density in the time available.

Anterior and posterior views of the chest, abdomen and pelvis are necessary since these aid the determination of the precise location of abnormal concentrations of the radiopharmaceutical. The normal body anatomy is clearly identifiable after ^{123}I has been used and body markers are generally not required. However, ^{137}Ba markers are valuable for anatomical orientation after ^{131}I-mIBG has been used, since the soft-tissue background activity which usually gives a body outline may not be sufficient for pinpointing lesions.

By convention, imaging is performed at 4 and 24 hours after administration of ^{123}I-mIBG, although the preliminary results of a study which we have carried out indicate that although imaging at 4 hours identifies most lesions, a small percentage may not be identified until 24 hours when the background activity has decreased. No lesions were identified at 4 hours alone, and therefore imaging at a single point in time, 24 hours, may be adequate. If the ^{131}I isotope has been used, imaging is usually performed at 24, 48 and 72 hours after administration of the radiopharmaceutical. Again most tumours are visible at 24 hours; however, the decline in liver activity may allow optimal imaging at 48 or 72 hours. Delayed imaging up to 7 days after injection permits assessment of ^{131}I-mIBG retention by the tumour for dosimetric calculations.

Table 3.2 summarises the projections, the length of time required for the acquisition of the images, and the timing of the images after administration of the radiopharmaceutical.

Single-photon Emission Computed Tomography

Emission tomography is particularly valuable in situations where the lesion is seen in an area of increased activity relative to the background level of radioactivity. The effect of tomography is to enhance the contrast between the levels of radioactivity making the lesion more obvious; in addition, the slice enables areas of overlapping

Table 3.2. Planar imaging

Isotope	Acquisition time per image	Time after injection	Projections
^{123}I	10 minutes	4 and 24 hours	Right lateral skull and arm Left lateral skull and arm Anterior chest Posterior chest
^{131}I	20 minutes	24, 48 and 72 hours	Anterior abdomen Posterior abdomen Anterior pelvis Posterior pelvis Anterior or posterior legs

activity on the planar views to be clearly separated. The time for which a patient can lie still may determine the total time of rotation, while the absorbed radiation dose determines the total activity which can be injected. The number of photons collected are always below the optimum level. Therefore the data must be processed to retain maximum detail while at the same time reducing mottle to a minimum. In spite of the restrictions imposed by the use of limited activities of radioisotope, there is no doubt that emission tomography improves the diagnostic sensitivity of ^{123}I-mIBG imaging. From phantom experiments we have found that the most useful measurements are those taken at 360° rotation in a series of 64 images, each acquired for 20 seconds. Reconstruction is carried out with a Ramp Hanning filter with a cut-off at a spatial frequency of $0.7 \, cm^{-1}$. The images are displayed in a 64×64 matrix using the transaxial, coronal and sagittal planes.

Hard Copy

All images are acquired as analogue images on film, and simultaneously in digital form as a 64×64 word-mode matrix for SPECT, and 128×128 word-mode matrix for planar imaging. Most information can be obtained by assessing the images interactively on the display monitor, varying the window levels to make the normal and abnormal activities most obvious. The system is set up so that the recorded images match those on the monitor. However, the comparison of the display monitor and the resulting image on film should be compared as part of the routine quality control.

In mIBG imaging the detail outlined above is especially necessary to ensure that sequential images taken during the course of the disease can be compared to follow changes in the size of the lesions and the levels of uptake in them.

4 Normal Pattern of Distribution of mIBG in Children with a History of Cancer

The normal distribution of mIBG which will be described relates to mIBG which has been radio-labelled with[123]I or [131]I. The occasions when there is an apparent difference in the sites of distribution between the two isotopes will be described separately.

As already discussed, ^{123}I-mIBG offers great advantages over ^{131}I-mIBG for imaging with modern gamma cameras. It has a lower photon energy which is more easily collimated; this, together with the increased photon flux, results in greater resolution and detail, and therefore it is more efficient at detecting lesions. The decay of ^{123}I is by electron capture, with minimal particulate emissions. This means that the radiation dose is less with [123]I. Thus 370 MBq (10 mCi) of ^{123}I-mIBG delivers approximately the same radiation absorbed dose as 18 MBq (0.5 mCi) ^{131}I-mIBG.

In the following chapters the term *I-mIGB will be used to denote mIBG which is radiolabelled with either the ^{123}I or ^{131}I isotope, unless it is specifically stated otherwise.

Normal Distribution

The patient population which we have studied to elucidate the normal (non-pathological) uptake of *I-mIBG includes children who had previously been diagnosed as having neuroblastoma, and in whom *I-mIBG studies had been performed when they had no evidence of disease as demonstrated by a variety of techniques (radiological, histological and bio-chemical). There was also a group of children who were initially thought to have neuroblastoma and therefore underwent mIBG scintigraphy, but who on subsequent investigations were shown to have tumours of non-neuroendocrine origin. (However, in order to illustrate certain anatomical points some of the images displayed in this chapter were obtained from patients with active neuroendocrine tumours.)

The sites where mIBG uptake was seen in these children included the thyroid gland, adrenal gland, heart, liver, spleen, kidneys and bladder, small and large bowel, salivary glands and lacrimal glands. Uptake of mIBG into these areas was regarded as non-pathological. Any foci of mIBG uptake other than into these organs or areas, were regarded as possible sites of neuroblastoma – either primary sites or metastatic sites of disease. It is interesting to note that mIBG is not taken up by the neurons of the central nervous system as it is thought not to cross the blood–brain barrier (Wieland et al. 1980).

The Thyroid Gland

Faint thyroid gland uptake of free ^{123}I or ^{131}I, which is mainly derived from in-vivo de-iodination, may be observed despite the use of various blocking regimens (Appendix D). In our series of patients, some thyroid uptake was seen in up to 60% of cases after the ^{123}I isotope had been used, and 10% of cases after the ^{131}I isotope had been used.

In Fig. 4.1.i the thyroid gland is seen particularly well. This child had refused to take her thyroid-blocking medication, resulting in the uptake of ^{123}I in the thyroid.

After targetted radiotherapy with ^{131}I-mIBG, thyroidal uptake of free ^{131}I occurred in more than 80% cases. In Fig. 4.1.ii the thyroid gland is again seen. This patient had received 5.4 GBq ^{131}I-mIBG for targetted radiotherapy 6 days previously. His thyroid had been blocked with appropriate oral medication which had been started 48 hours before the ^{131}I-mIBG was given.

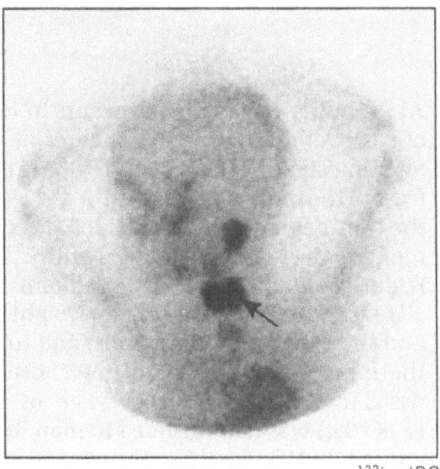

^{123}I-mIBG

^{131}I-mIBG

24 hours

Fig. 4.1.i. Left lateral skull. An unblocked thyroid gland showing intense concentration of ^{123}I (*arrow*) because the patient did not take the prescribed Lugol's iodine.

6 days

Fig. 4.1.ii. Left lateral skull. Thyroid gland uptake is clearly seen (*arrow*) in this patient after a therapeutic dose of ^{131}I-mIBG had been given, despite taking Lugol's iodine 0.2 ml p.o. t.d.s as prescribed.

The Adrenal Gland

The highest uptake and most prolonged retention of mIBG occurs in the adrenal medulla. In vitro incubation studies using bovine adrenal medullary cells or human phaeochromocytoma cells in culture have shown that ^{125}I-mIBG and ^{3}H-noradrenaline share similar specific, active, energy- and sodium-dependent uptake mechanisms (Jaques et al. 1984). As well as sharing the same uptake pathway they also compete with each other for it. Uptake of mIBG by the adrenal medulla and sympathetic autonomic neurons occurs by two processes: a specific active process known as type I uptake and a non-specific, concentration-dependent passive diffusional process known as type 2 uptake.

The type 1 uptake is a sodium-dependent pump which is temperature sensitive, and is also characterised by high-affinity, low-capacity, saturability. It may be inhibited by desmethylimipramine and cocaine. Once taken up, the mIBG is stored in the intracellular hormone/neurotransmitter storage granules of the sympathomedullary tissues. Thus the scintigraphic distribution of mIBG reflects the specific and non-specific uptake and storage capacity of the radiopharmaceutical. High-performance liquid chromatography (HPLC) of extracts of human phaeochromocytoma labelled preoperatively with ^{131}I-mIBG shows that the radiopharmaceutical is taken up and stored as unaltered ^{131}I-mIBG (Mangner et al. 1986).

The normal adrenal medulla is not usually visualised by ^{131}I-mIBG using standard diagnostic doses.

At 24 hours visible uptake occurs in less than 10% of cases, and in only 16% of cases at 48–72 hours after injection (Nakajo et al. 1983a). This is in contrast to the reports of Wieland et al. (1980) in which the normal adrenal glands of dogs and rhesus monkeys were readily imaged with ^{131}I-mIBG. This is due to a difference in the administered dose of ^{131}I-mIBG per kilogram of body weight given to man and the experimental animals, and to the fact that the human adrenal gland has considerably more tissue overlying it. An average of 0.26 MBq/kg (7 μCi/kg) was administered to man, in comparison with 2.22 MBq/kg (60 μCi/kg) and 4.81 MBq/kg (130 μCi/kg) to dogs and monkeys respectively. The adrenal medulla is regularly depicted when doses of 75–370 MBq (2–10 mCi) are used. Adrenal gland uptake may be quantified in vivo and has been estimated to be 0.01% to 0.3% of the administered dose at 22 hours (Bomanji et al. 1986).

Scintigraphy with ^{123}I-mIBG routinely visualises the normal adrenal medulla, and we have found that both adrenal glands are seen regularly on the 4-hour study, but may not be seen on the 24-hour study. The left adrenal gland is seen more often than the right, but this may be due to the fact that the right adrenal gland is situated close to the liver which masks the uptake in the adrenal area.

Figures 4.2.i–v show three different patients who all show good uptake of ^{123}I-mIBG in the left adrenal, but the right adrenal is more difficult to see due to its close proximity to the liver.

On opposite page

Fig. 4.2.i. Posterior chest and abdomen. This child has neuro-blastoma and the left adrenal gland is clearly seen (*arrow*).

Fig. 4.2.ii. Posterior chest and abdomen. The left adrenal gland is clearly seen (*arrow*), and the pelves of both kidneys (*arrows*) show increased activity, due to the excretion of mIBG via the kidneys.

Fig. 4.2.iii. Posterior chest and abdomen (same patient as in Fig. 4.2.ii). The left adrenal gland is again clearly seen (*arrow*), and the activity previously seen in the right renal pelvis is no longer visible. This child also has uptake into a soft-tissue site of ganglioneuroma in the left side of the chest, superior to the heart (*arrow*).

Fig. 4.2.iv. Posterior abdomen. The left adrenal gland is again clearly visualised (*arrow*) in this patient who has a malignant phaeochromocytoma. A site of increased uptake of mIBG which corresponds to a lesion in a lumber vertebral body (*arrow*) is also well seen.

Fig. 4.2.v. Posterior abdomen (same patient as in Fig. 4.2.iv. The left adrenal gland is again well seen (*arrow*), and the right adrenal gland can also be delineated (*arrow*).

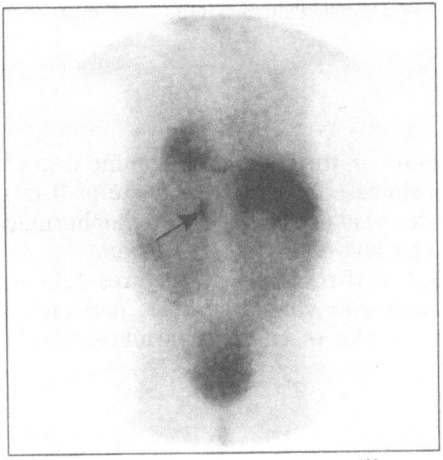

¹²³I-mIBG

24 hours

Fig. 4.2.i. Posterior chest and abdomen.

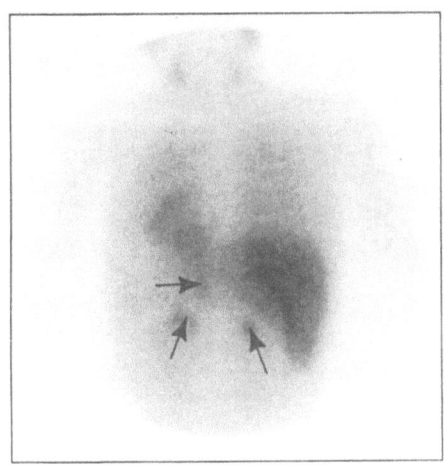

¹²³I-mIBG

4 hours

Fig. 4.2.ii. Posterior chest and abdomen.

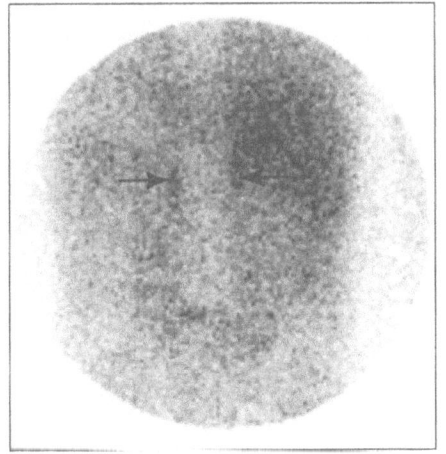

¹²³I-mIBG

24 hours

Fig. 4.2.iii. Posterior chest and abdomen (same patient as in Fig. 4.2.ii).

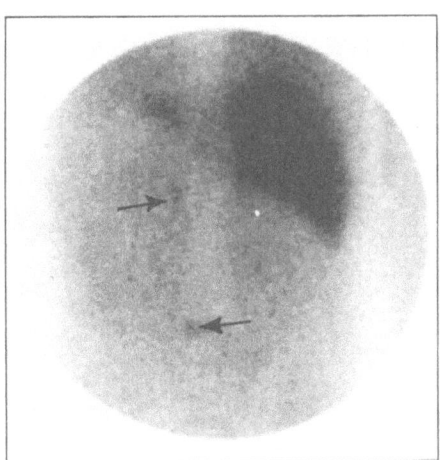

¹²³I-mIBG

4 hours

Fig. 4.2.iv. Posterior abdomen.

¹²³I-mIBG

24 hours

Fig. 4.2.v. Posterior abdomen (same patient as in Fig. 4.2.iv).

25

The Liver

The organ with the greatest uptake is the liver, despite the fact that in animal studies the concentration of ^{125}I-mIBG in the liver was only 1.5 and 2 times that in the blood at 24 and 48 hours respectively (Nakajo et al. 1983a). It is routinely seen and this is probably a reflection of its volume and vascularity. It is also a major site of catecholamine degradation, and therefore it may also be a site of *I-mIBG uptake, even though most of the radiopharmaceutical is excreted unchanged in the urine.

Figures 4.3.i–ii are ^{123}I-mIBG scintigrams of the same patient, showing uptake of the radiopharmaceutical into the liver.

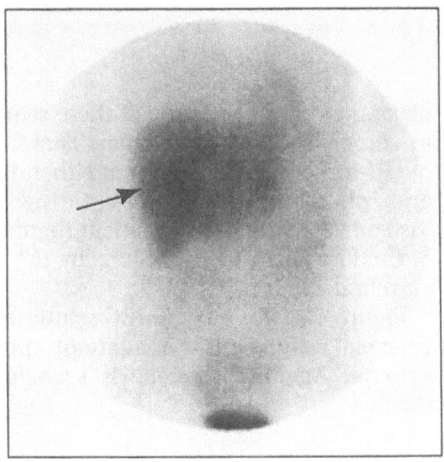
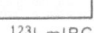

¹²³I-mIBG

4 hours

Fig. 4.3.i. Posterior abdomen. The liver shows intense uptake of ^{123}I-mIBG (*arrow*).

¹²³I-mIBG

24 hours

Fig. 4.3.ii. Posterior abdomen (same patient as in Fig. 4.3.i). The activity in the liver has diminished at 24 hours.

The Spleen

Splenic uptake is seen in most studies, the level increasing with time after administration of the mIBG (Nakajo et al. 1983a). This is the reverse of that observed in the liver, and the reason is thought to lie with the spleen's rich sympathetic innervation. Our experience is that there is little splenic uptake in children, and in fact often a photon–deficient area is seen at the site of the spleen.

Figures 4.4.i–ii show ^{123}I-mIBG scintigrams taken at 4 and 24 hours in the same patient. This child had previously been diagnosed as having neuro-blastoma, but at the time of these scintigrams was in complete clinical remission. There is no uptake of ^{123}I-mIBG into the spleen at either 4 or 24 hours and photon-deficient areas (arrows) are seen instead. Note that in this patient there is absorption of the low-energy ^{123}I photons by the bones of the vertebral column.

Figure 4.4.iii is a ^{123}I-mIBG scintigram of an 18-year-old male with malignant phaeochromo-cytoma. Again no uptake is seen in the spleen (arrow).

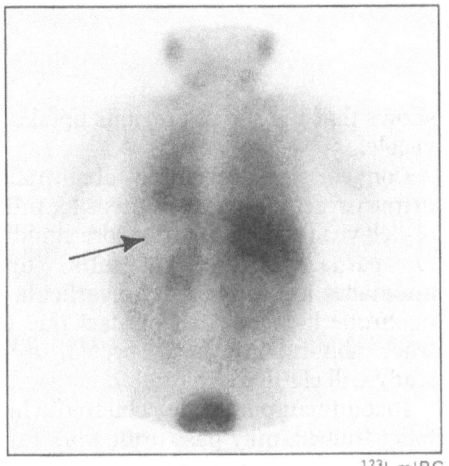

¹²³I-mIBG

4 hours

Fig. 4.4.i. Posterior abdomen. The spleen (*arrow*) is seen as a photon-deficient area.

¹²³I-mIBG

24 hours

Fig. 4.4.ii. Posterior abdomen (same patient as in Fig. 4.4.i). At 24 hours, there is still no uptake into the spleen (*arrow*).

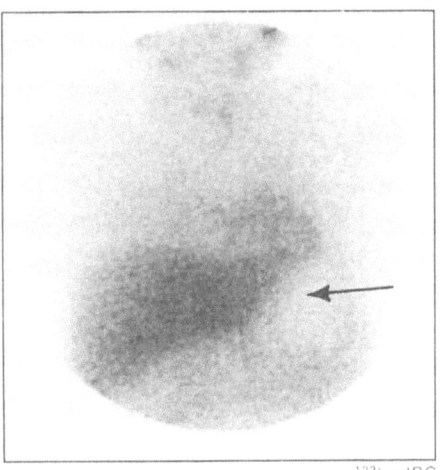

¹²³I-mIBG

24 hours

Fig. 4.4.iii. Anterior chest. This patient has a malignant phaeochromocytoma and shows no splenic uptake (*arrow*).

The Kidneys and Bladder

The mIBG is excreted via the urinary tract, with about 60% being eliminated in the first 24 hours. Occasionally the kidneys are visualised at 24 hours, but rarely later due to the rapid renal clearance of *I-mIBG. The presence of *I-mIBG in the urine results in the regular visualisation of the urinary bladder, and the intensity of bladder visualisation declines with time. Excretion of *I-mIBG is reduced in patients with impaired renal function, a factor which should be considered when embarking on mIBG therapy.

The urinary excretion of mIBG means that care has to be taken to exclude urinary contamination as the cause of uptake. In Fig. 4.5.i a spot of urine on the skin of the left side of the neck (arrow) could have been mistaken for an involved lymph node in this child with neuroblastoma. A repeat examination at 24 hours (Fig. 4.5.ii) in the same patient shows that the site of previous uptake is no longer visible.

Congenital or acquired abnormalities of the urinary tract may provide areas for mIBG retention or delayed transit, and therefore could be mistaken for pathological foci of mIBG uptake. Such anomalies include bladder diverticula or a hydronephrotic kidney. If an artefact due to a urinary tract abnormality is suspected, a ^{99m}Tc-DTPA study will clarify the situation.

Incontinent patients or children who are not yet toilet-trained, may pass urine into a nappy during the scanning procedure (Fig. 4.5.iii). Should this occur, a scintigram of the contaminated area should be repeated after the nappy has been changed and the napkin area cleaned. This is essential to avoid false positive or false negative studies.

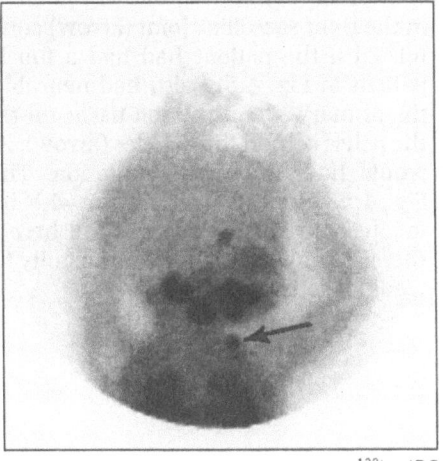

123I-mIBG

4 hours

Fig. 4.5.i. Right lateral skull. Urine contamination on the left side of the neck (*arrow*) could be mistaken for pathological soft tissue uptake.

123I-mIBG

24 hours

Fig. 4.5.ii. Right lateral skull (same patient as in Fig. 4.5.i). Following decontamination the 'lesion' is no longer visible.

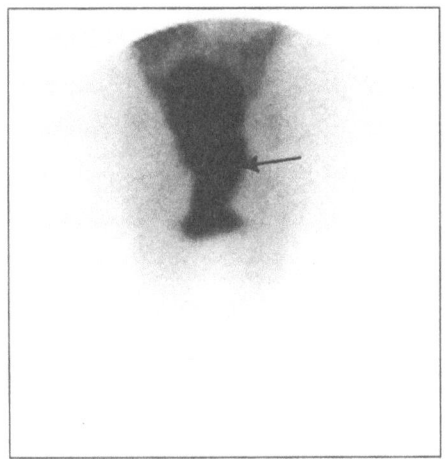

123I-mIBG

4 hours

Fig. 4.5.iii. Anterior pelvis. Urine contamination into a nappy (*arrow*), resulting in an uninformative mIBG scintigram (see text).

continued

Since mIBG is excreted by the kidneys it is important to scan the abdomen and pelvis when the patient has an empty bladder, if possible. In the infant this may be difficult and therefore, if it is thought that a lesion may be masked by activity in the bladder, catheterisation of the child should be considered prior to scintigraphy. Figures 4.5.iv–vi demonstrate the importance of this. The patient in Fig. 4.5.iv had widespread neuroblastoma with bone marrow and focal bone involvement. A lesion in the right sacroiliac joint (arrow) could have been missed if the patient had had a full bladder. The patient in Fig. 4.5.v also had neuroblastoma with the primary site in the soft tissue on the left side of the pelvis behind the bladder (arrow). A full bladder would have obscured this lesion. The patient in Fig. 4.5.vi had neuroblastoma with bone marrow involvement. The bladder is full here (arrow) and therefore any lesion in close proximity to the bladder would be missed.

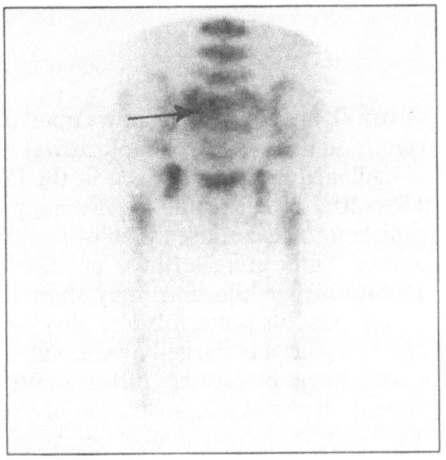

¹²³I-mIBG

24 hours

Fig. 4.5.iv. Posterior pelvis. The importance of scanning with an empty bladder is well shown in this patient with widespread neuroblastoma involving the bone marrow and cortical bone. The lesion in the left sacroiliac joint (*arrow*) would have been more difficult to see if the bladder had been full.

¹²³I-mIBG

24 hours

Fig. 4.5.v. Posterior pelvis. The importance of scanning with an empty bladder is again demonstrated in this patient with stage IV neuroblastoma. The primary site is in the soft tissue (*arrow*) in the left hemi-pelvis behind the bladder. There is also obvious bone marrow involvement.

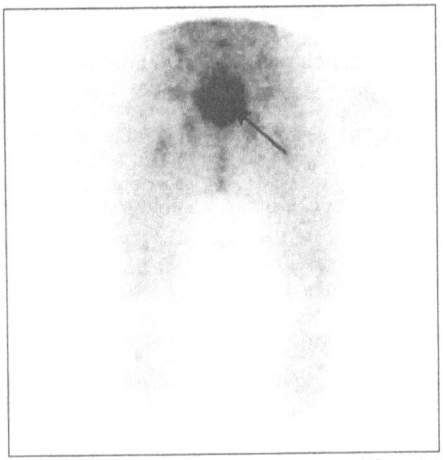

¹²³I-mIBG

24 hours

Fig. 4.5.vi. Posterior pelvis. In this patient with stage IV neuroblastoma involving the bone marrow, any lesion lying in close relation to the bladder (*arrow*) would have been obscured by the activity in the urine contained there.

The Gastrointestinal Tract

*I-mIBG is normally seen in the small and large bowel. The mechanism by which it reaches the bowel lumen is not clear. In a study of guanethidine distribution in the rat, 8% of the intravenous dose was excreted in the faeces by 18 hours via biliary excretion, pancreatic excretion, and direct passage across the gastrointestinal epithelium (Nakajo et al. 1983a). Since *I-mIBG is an analogué of guanethidine, it may also be similarly excreted. Another possible route is from the ingestion of saliva which has been shown to contain excreted mIBG radioactivity. There may also be uptake via autonomic neuronal elements into the bowel wall itself.

Figures 4.6.i–iii show ^{123}I-mIBG scintigrams illustrating radioactivity within the lumen or wall of the intestine. In Fig. 4.6.i uptake is seen in the ascending colon (arrows) in a patient with neuroblastoma and abdominal para-aortic node relapse. Figure 4.6.ii shows uptake in the transverse colon (arrows), and Fig. 4.6.iii shows uptake in the transverse and descending colon (arrows).

Radioactivity may be seen in the large bowel in 15%–20% of cases and occasionally this may be sufficient to be confused with or to obscure tumour uptake. Early images (those acquired at less than 18 hours after injection) may show loops of small bowel, but this pattern is less obvious at 24 hours and is replaced by large-bowel uptake.

We have performed mIBG scintigraphy in a patient after oral administration of ^{123}I-mIBG (Figs. 4.6.iv–v). There was similar uptake of mIBG within known tumour sites (both with respect to anatomical location and intensity of uptake), to that which had been seen after intravenous injection of ^{123}I-mIBG. However oral *I-mIBG does result in increased radioactivity in the gastrointestinal tract, and this of course could obscure lesions in or close to the bowel.

On opposite page

Fig. 4.6.i. Anterior abdomen and pelvis. Uptake is seen in the ascending colon (*arrows*) in this patient with neuroblastoma with para-aortic nodal relapse.

Fig. 4.6.ii. Anterior chest and abdomen. Uptake is seen in the transverse colon (*arrows*).

Fig. 4.6.iii. Anterior abdomen and pelvis. Uptake is seen in the transverse and descending colon (*arrows*).

Fig. 4.6.iv. Anterior chest and abdomen. This scintigram was performed after oral administration of 185 MBq of ^{123}I-mIBG. Increased uptake is seen in the transverse colon (*arrows*).

Fig. 4.6.v. Anterior abdomen and pelvis (same patient as in Fig. 4.6.iv). This shows good uptake of mIBG into the ascending and descending colon (*arrows*: *ac, dc*) and also into the sites of the tumour (*arrows*: *t*).

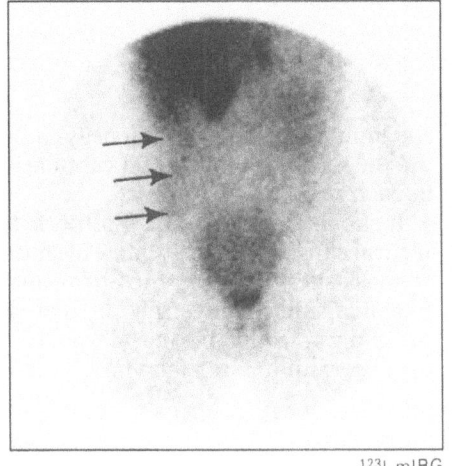

24 hours

Fig. 4.6.i. Anterior abdomen and pelvis.

Fig. 4.6.ii. Anterior chest and abdomen.

24 hours

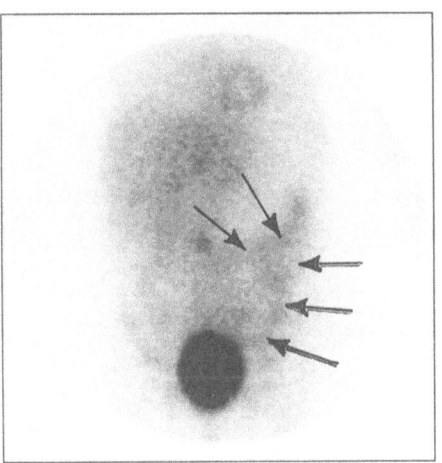

24 hours

Fig. 4.6.iii: Anterior abdomen and pelvis.

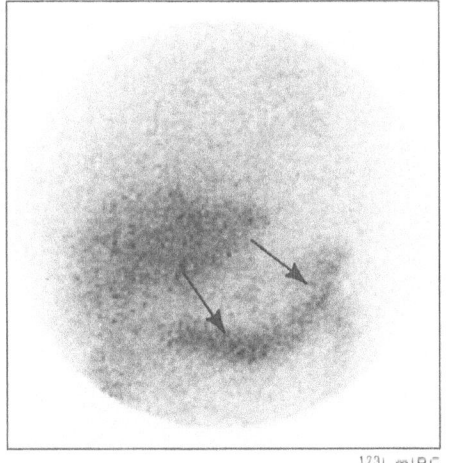

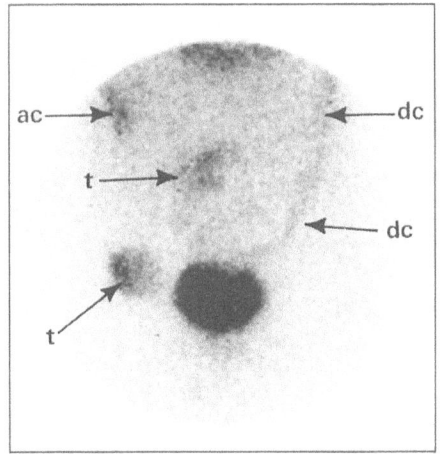

24 hours

Fig. 4.6.iv. Anterior chest and abdomen.

24 hours

Fig. 4.6.v. Anterior abdomen and pelvis (same patient as in Fig. 4.6.iv).

35

The Lung

The lung shows high uptake immediately after and for about 4 hours following injection (Fig. 4.7.i). This concentration of *I-mIBG may be a non-specific diffusional uptake by endothelial cells due to the high initial concentration of *I-mIBG presented to the lung. There is a rapid fall in lung activity, with little being detected at 24 hours (Fig. 4.7.ii), and therefore this uptake is unlikely to interfere with interpretation of the scintigrams. Uptake in each of the lung zones varies in intensity, probably reflecting the relative volumes and vascularity of the lung in each zone.

It should be noted that *I-mIBG is taken up into pleural effusions (Fig. 4.7.iii). This has the potential to mask sites of disease thereby resulting in a false negative study. Conversely, increased uptake into an effusion could be misinterpreted as a site of disease, resulting in a false positive study.

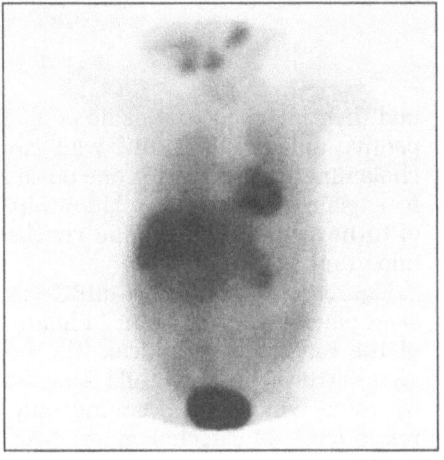

¹²³I-mIBG

4 hours

Fig. 4.7.i. Anterior chest and abdomen. Increased uptake of mIBG is seen in both lungs at 4 hours after injection of the radiopharmaceutical, in comparison with the uptake seen in Fig. 4.7.ii which was obtained 24 hours after injection.

¹²³I-mIBG

24 hours

Fig. 4.7.ii. Anterior chest and abdomen. After 24 hours the lung activity is greatly reduced.

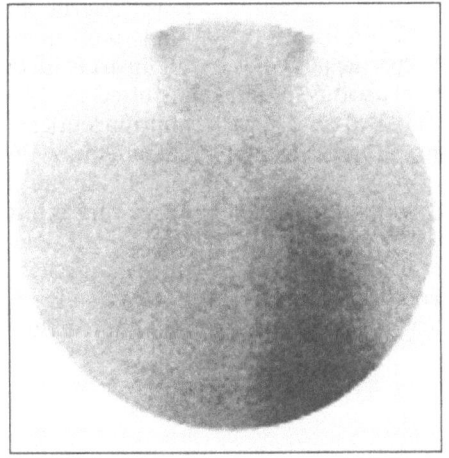

¹²³I-mIBG

24 hours

Fig. 4.7.iii. Posterior chest. ¹²³I-mIBG in a left-sided pleural effusion.

The Heart

Visualisation of the myocardium with *I-mIBG is variable. All four chambers of the heart have a rich sympathetic innervation, and its ability to rapidly concentrate ^{3}H-noradrenaline has been well documented (Crout 1964). Although 80% of the noradrenaline present in the heart is synthesised there, the myocardium can avidly accumulate exogenous noradrenaline. In adrenergic nerve endings mIBG shares the same uptake, storage and release mechanisms as noradrenaline, but is metabolised differently and therefore its transit time may be delayed.

The high levels of ^{123}I-mIBG image the heart clearly. Catecholamines are taken up by the heart into several compartments, of which two are the most important. The first is a neuronal compartment dependent on the uptake 1 mechanism, and inhibited by cocaine, reserpine and desimipramine. The second is a group of non-neuronal compartments that are dependent on the uptake 2 mechanism, and may be inhibited by phenoxybenzamine, normetadrenaline and steroid hormones. Non-neuronal uptake of *I-mIBG in the heart is observed only at very low specific activities. The radio-iodinated mIBG in general use has specific activities of 37–3700 MBq/kg (1–100 mCi/mg), and therefore in man the neuronal uptake usually predominates.

It has been hypothesised that prevailing levels of catecholamines in plasma might influence *I-mIBG uptake by the heart, and it has been shown that an inverse relationship exists between visualisation of the heart and plasma and urinary catecholamines

and their metabolites (Nakajo et al. 1983b). Competitive uptake of *I-mIBG with circulating catecholamines in the heart is one possible mechanism to explain this inverse relationship, but rapidity of turnover of noradrenaline vesicles may also be important.

Figures 4.8.i–ii show ^{123}I-mIBG scintigrams of the same patient taken at 4 and 24 hours after injection of the radiopharmaceutical. The heart is clearly seen (arrows) in this child who had a ganglioneuroma which was secreting only very slightly raised levels of catecholamines. This is in marked contrast to the patient illustrated in Figs. 4.8.iii–iv, who had a malignant phaeochromocytoma and was secreting very high levels of catecholamines. The heart does not appear to take up mIBG and in fact is seen as a photon-deficient area (arrows). The child illustrated in Fig. 4.8.v had neuroblastoma with an abdominal para-aortic node relapse (arrow) which is clearly seen lying inferior and medial to the lower lateral border of the liver. He was secreting moderately increased levels of catecholamines, and the heart is just visible in this ^{131}I-mIBG scintigram acquired at 24 hours after injection of the radiopharmaceutical.

Sometimes the heart may not be seen, and this may be due to the simultaneous administration of drugs that interfere with the uptake of *I-mIBG by the heart, such as reserpine, tricyclic antidepressants, and phenylpropanolamine. Cardiac uptake is also reduced in autonomic neuropathy, and immediately following myocardial infarction.

On opposite page

Fig. 4.8.i. Posterior chest and abdomen. Good uptake is seen within the heart (*arrow*) in this child with a ganglioneuroma and who was secreting marginally raised levels of catecholamines.

Fig. 4.8.ii. Posterior chest and abdomen (same patient as in Fig. 4.8.i).

Fig. 4.8.iii. Anterior chest. A photon-deficient area is seen at the site of the heart (*arrow*) in this patient with a malignant phaeochromocytoma who was secreting markedly raised levels of catecholamines.

Fig. 4.8.iv. Anterior chest (same patient as in Fig. 4.8.iii).

Fig. 4.8.v. Anterior chest and abdomen. The heart is only just seen (*arrow*) in this child with a relapse of neuroblastoma in the para-aortic area, who was secreting moderately raised levels of catecholamines.

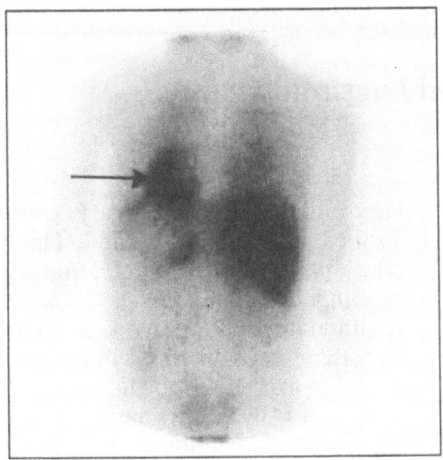

4 hours

Fig. 4.8.i. Posterior chest and abdomen.

^{123}I-mIBG

24 hours

Fig. 4.8.ii. Posterior chest and abdomen (same patient as in Fig. 4.8.i).

^{123}I-mIBG

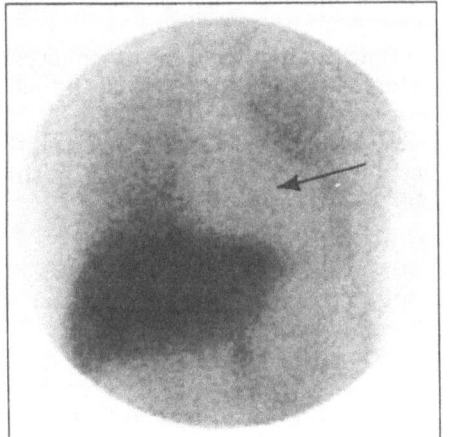

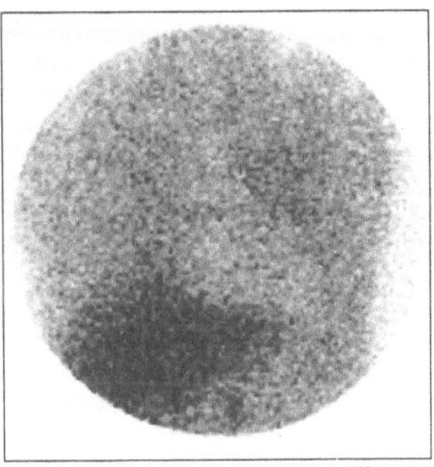

4 hours

Fig. 4.8.iii. Anterior chest.

^{123}I-mIBG

24 hours

Fig. 4.8.iv. Anterior chest (same patient as in Fig. 4.8.iii).

^{123}I-mIBG

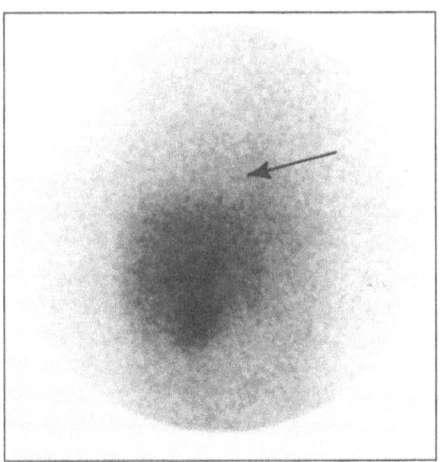

24 hours

Fig. 4.8.v. Anterior chest and abdomen.

^{131}I-mIBG

The Salivary Glands, Nasopharynx and Lacrimal Glands

The salivary glands are particularly well-delineated in mIBG examinations. From studies in animals and man it has been shown that the mechanism of salivary gland uptake of *I-mIBG is not a simple glandular concentration of radioiodide. The discrepancy between salivary gland and gastric visualisation suggests a specific uptake of *I-mIBG. This *I-mIBG uptake by the salivary glands is neuronal as shown by studies in dogs. These have demonstrated that ^{131}I-mIBG is present equally in the submandibular and parotid glands, both of which are innervated by the sympathetic nervous system, although only the parotid gland is able to concentrate iodide. The neuronal nature of the *I-mIBG uptake is further suggested by the inhibition of such uptake by tricylic antidepressants, the lack of *I-mIBG uptake by the salivary glands in a patient suffering from severe autonomic neuropathy, and also the ipsilateral decrease in *I-mIBG uptake by the salivary glands of a patient with specific adrenergic sympathetic denervation of these glands due to surgically induced Horner's syndrome (Nakajo et al. 1984).

Figure 4.9.i shows salivary gland uptake of ^{123}I-mIBG (arrows) in a child. Fig. 4.9.ii shows similar uptake into the parotid and submandibular glands in a teenager.

Additional studies have also shown that the radioactivity seen in the salivary glands on scintigraphy is excreted into the saliva. Although the secretion of saliva is primarily governed by parasympathetic innervation of the salivary glands, the sympathetic nervous system modulates the composition of the saliva secreted. Of the radioactivity in the saliva, 98% is free ^{131}I while 2% is ^{131}I-labelled mIBG. This excretion of radioactivity represents only a small fraction of the total activity in the gland.

The visualisation of the nasopharynx (Fig. 4.9.ii) is thought to occur as a result of its rich sympathetic innervation.

When the ^{123}I isotope is used there is faint lacrimal uptake which is clearly shown in Figs. 4.9.iii–iv (arrows).

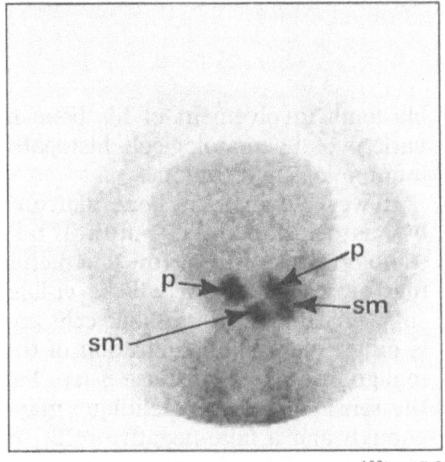

^{123}I-mIBG

24 hours

Fig. 4.9.i. Right lateral skull. Good uptake is seen in the parotid glands (*arrows: p*) and submandibular glands (*arrows: sm*).

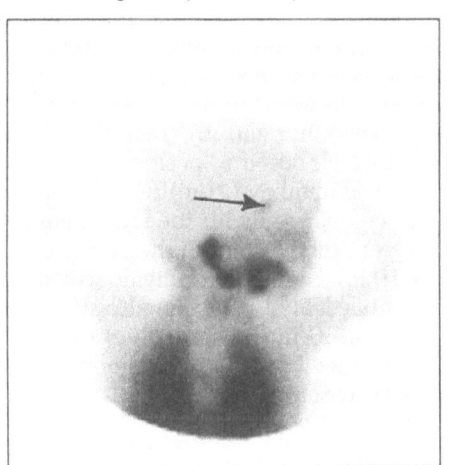

^{123}I-mIBG

4 hours

Fig. 4.9.ii. Anterior skull. Good uptake is again seen in the salivary glands (*arrows*) and the nasopharynx (*arrow np*).

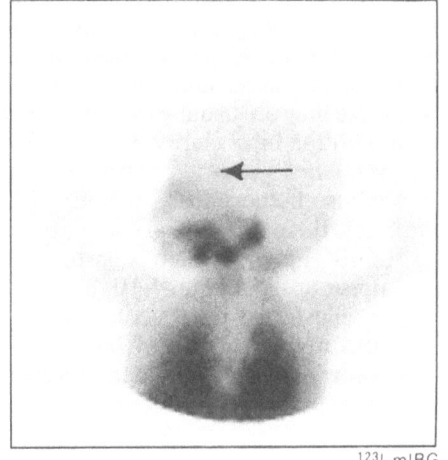

^{123}I-mIBG

4 hours

Fig. 4.9.iii. Right lateral skull. Uptake is seen in the lacrimal glands (*arrow*).

^{123}I-mIBG

4 hours

Fig. 4.9.iv. Left lateral skull. Uptake is seen in the left lacrimal gland (*arrow*); this is usually no longer visible at 24 hours after injection of the radiopharmaceutical.

The Bone Marrow

Before proceeding to discuss the variation in normal scintigram appearances obtained after administration of either ^{123}I-mIBG or ^{131}I-mIBG, the appearances of normal bone and infiltrated bone and bone marrow should be considered. For the purposes of mIBG scintigraphy, bone can be considered as an outer hard cortex and an inner central "hollow" compartment containing the bone marrow. When neuroblastoma spreads from its site of origin it may infiltrate the bone marrow or the cortical bone, either separately or together. On mIBG scintigraphy normal bone and bone marrow do not take up *I-mIBG, and therefore cannot be distinguished from the diffuse background activity.

The bones that contain the most active functional bone marrow are the long bones of the arms and legs, the pelvis and the vertebral column. Figs 4.10.i–vi illustrate a patient with and without bone marrow involvement by neuroblastoma. To assess whether the bone marrow is infiltrated by tumour the long bones of the arms and legs should be examined first since they are usually the sites which demonstrate it with the most clarity. In Fig. 4.10.i and Fig. 4.10.v the arms and legs can be seen to have either a diffuse homogeneous pattern of *I-mIBG uptake across them or a central compartment of decreased *I-mIBG uptake (which is particularly evident in the upper arms). In Fig. 4.10.iii the vertebral column is illustrated by a vertical strip of decreased *I-mIBG uptake. Figures 4.10.i, iii and v are scintigrams which were obtained when the patient was shown to have no evidence of neuro-blastoma involvement of his bone marrow by a variety of haematological, histopathological and immunological techniques.

However, when the bone marrow is infiltrated by neuroblastoma, the *I-mIBG is taken up by the tumour cells in the marrow and therefore the bone-marrow compartment will be visible if there are sufficient numbers of tumour cells present. If there is only a very light infiltration of the marrow by malignant cells, as in Case 3 (see Figs 5.3.v–viii), the sensitivity of the technique may not be good enough and a false-negative mIBG result may be obtained. In our experience this is very unusual, and mIBG scintigraphy as a single investigation has been extremely sensitive at predicting bone marrow infiltration by neuroblastoma. Figures 4.10.ii, iv and vi illustrate widespread bone marrow infiltration by neuroblastoma at the proximal ends of the central compartments of both humera and femora. Characteristically, the proximal ends of the long bones show *I-mIBG uptake when there is bone-marrow invasion by neuroblastoma, before the distal ends become "positive". Figure 4.10.iv shows intense uptake of *I-mIBG in the vertebral column (in comparison with the low-intensity vertical strip seen at the position of the vertebral column in Fig. 4.10.iii), and the individual vertebrae can be identified. Figure 4.10.vi also shows intense uptake of *I-mIBG in the skeleton of the pelvis and in the iliac crests, which are common sites used for bone marrow sampling.

On opposite page

Fig. 4.10.i. Left lateral skull. Normal bone marrow of the skull and long bones of the arms.

Fig. 4.10.ii. Left lateral skull. Increased uptake is seen in the bone marrow of the humerus (see text above for more details).

Fig. 4.10.iii. Posterior chest and abdomen. No uptake of *I-mIBG is seen in the vertebral column.

Fig. 4.10.iv. Posterior chest and abdomen. Intense abnormal uptake of *I-mIBG is seen in individual vertebrae.

Fig. 4.10.v. Posterior abdomen and pelvis. No uptake of *I-mIBG is seen in the pelvis or the bone marrow of the femora.

Fig. 4.10.vi. Posterior abdomen and pelvis. Intense uptake of *I-mIBG is seen in the bone marrow of the femora. Uptake is also seen in the skeleton of the pelvis, which is also rich in bone marrow.

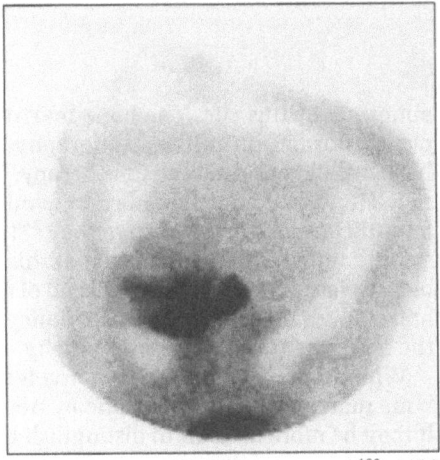

¹²³I-mIBG

24 hours
Fig. 4.10.i. Left lateral skull.

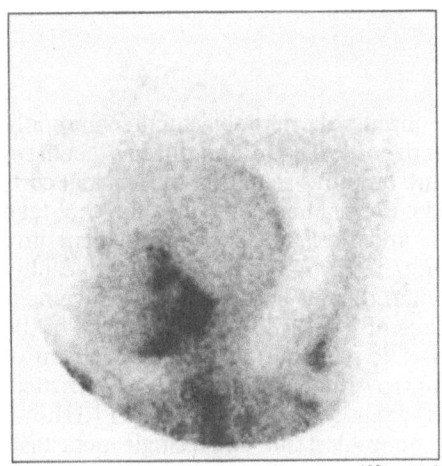

¹²³I-mIBG

24 hours
Fig. 4.10.ii. Left lateral skull.

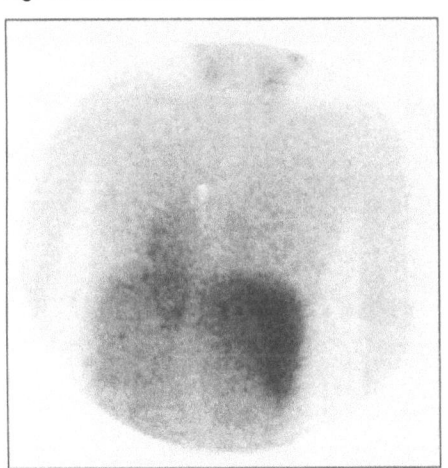

¹²³I-mIBG

24 hours
Fig. 4.10.iii. Posterior chest and abdomen.

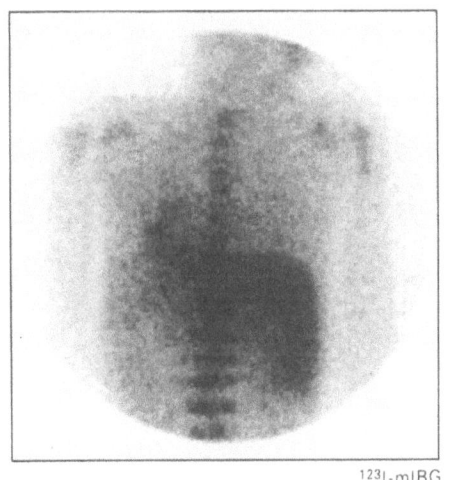

¹²³I-mIBG

24 hours
Fig. 4.10.iv. Posterior chest and abdomen.

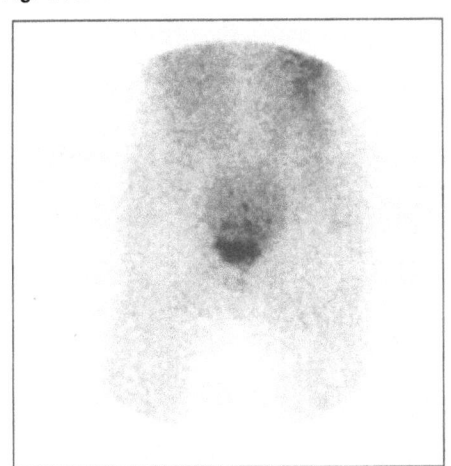

¹²³I-mIBG

24 hours
Fig. 4.10.v. Posterior abdomen and pelvis.

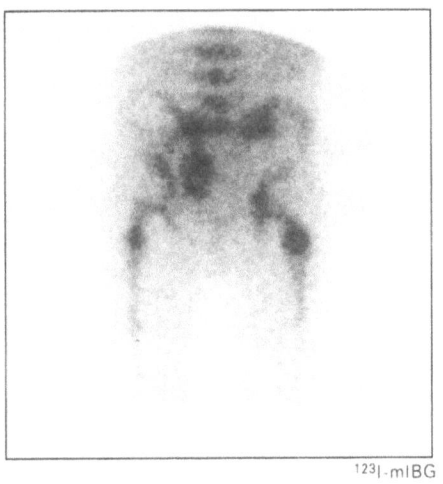

¹²³I-mIBG

24 hours
Fig. 4.10.vi. Posterior abdomen and pelvis.

Bone

As already discussed, neuroblastoma commonly metastasizes to cortical bone, and this has a characteristic picture on mIBG scintigraphy. Normal cortical bone (like normal bone marrow) does not take up *I-mIBG, and therefore does not present any distinguishing features on mIBG scintigraphy. However, when there is cortical bone involvement intense uptake of *I-mIBG is seen at the site of the lesion. If there is no simultaneous involvement of the bone marrow by neuroblastoma the cortical bone lesions are easily identifiable. Fig. 4.11.i shows a child with neuroblastoma and a single metastasis in the cortical bone of the lower third of the left femur. The ^{99m}Tc-MDP bone scintigram was also abnormal at this site. The bone marrow was completely normal on mIBG scintigraphy and also on histopathology. After chemotherapy, Fig. 4.11.ii now shows a completely normal femur on the left on mIBG scintigraphy, despite the ^{99m}Tc-MDP bone scintigram remaining abnormal at this site. A bone biopsy was taken from the distal end of the left femur and showed no evidence of malignancy, confirming the assessment by mIBG scintigraphy.

When there is simultaneous involvement of the bone marrow and cortical bone by neuroblastoma, it may be more difficult to distinguish the two components. Several illustrations of this point are demonstrated in the case studies in Chapter 5.

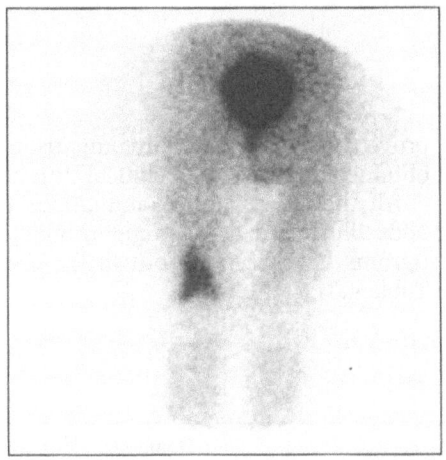

123I-mIBG   123I-mIBG

24 hours

Fig. 4.11.i. Posterior view of the legs. Intense uptake of mIBG is seen at the distal end of the left femur whilst the bone marrow of the femur is normal. A ^{99m}Tc-MDP bone scintigram was also abnormal at this site.

24 hours

Fig. 4.11.ii. Posterior view of the legs. The left femur appears normal now (^{99m}Tc-MDP bone scintigram was still abnormal). A biopsy at this site confirmed there was no disease.

Normal mIBG Studies in Children of Different Ages

The remainder of this chapter is devoted to illustrating the range of normal studies in different age groups (infant to teenager), obtained using both ^{123}I-mIBG and ^{131}I-mIBG. The images have been acquired at varying times after administration of the radiopharmaceutical. It is hoped that they will prove useful as a basis for comparison with images obtained in a variety of clinical situations.

All the studies are examinations of the whole body illustrated as overlapping images. The scintigrams have been set out in the order shown in Table 4.1.

Table 4.1. Display of scintigrams

	Radiopharmaceutical	Time	Figures
a.	^{123}I-mIBG	4 hours after intravenous ^{123}I-mIBG	4.12–4.15
b.	^{123}I-mIBG	24 hours after intravenous ^{123}I-mIBG	4.16–4.19
c.	^{131}I-mIBG	24 hours after intravenous ^{131}I-mIBG	4.20–4.23
d.	^{131}I-mIBG	48 hours after intravenous ^{131}I-mIBG	4.24–4.27
e.	^{131}I-mIBG	72 hours after intravenous ^{131}I-mIBG	4.28–4.31

References

Bomanji J, Flatman WO, Horne T et al. (1986) Quantitation of 123–I-metaiodobenzylguanidine (MIBG) uptake by normal adrenal medulla, Nucl Med Commun 7:296

Crout JR (1964) The uptake and release of ^{3}H-norepinephrine by the guinea pig heart in vivo, Arch Exp Pathol Pharmacol 248:85–98

Jaques S, Tobes MC, Sisson JC et al. (194) Comparison of the sodium dependency of uptake of meta-iodobenzylguanidine and norepinephrine into cultured bovine adrenomedullary cells, Molec Pharmacol 26:539–546

Mangner TJ, Tobes MC, Wieland DM et al. (1986) Metabolism of meta-I-131-iodobenzylguanidine in patients with metastatic phaeochromocytoma; concise communication, J Nucl Med 27:37–44

Nakajo M, Shapiro B, Copp J et al. (1983a) The normal and abnormal distribution of the adrenomedullary imaging agent m-[I-131]iodobenzylguanidine (I-131 MIBG) in man; evaluation by scintigraphy, J Nucl Med 24:672–682

Nakajo M, Shapiro B, Glowniak J et al. (1983b) Inverse relationship between cardiac accumulation of meta-[^{131}I]iodobenzylguanidine (I-131 MIGB) and circulating catecholamines in suspected phaeochromocytoma, J Nucl Med 24:1127–1134

Nakajo M, Shapiro B, Sisson JC et al. (1984) Salivary gland accumulation of meta-[^{131}I]iodobenzylguanidine, J Nucl Med 25:2–6

Wieland DM, Wu J-L, Brown LE et al. (1980) Radiolabeled adrenergic neuron-blocking agents; adrenomedullary imaging with [^{131}I]iodobenzylguanidine, J Nucl Med 21:349–353

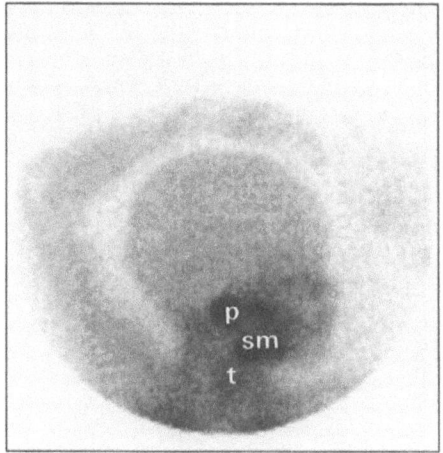

Fig. 4.12.i. Child: right lateral skull

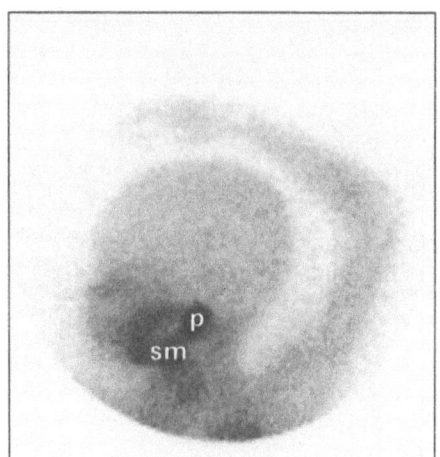

Fig. 4.12.ii. Child: left lateral skull

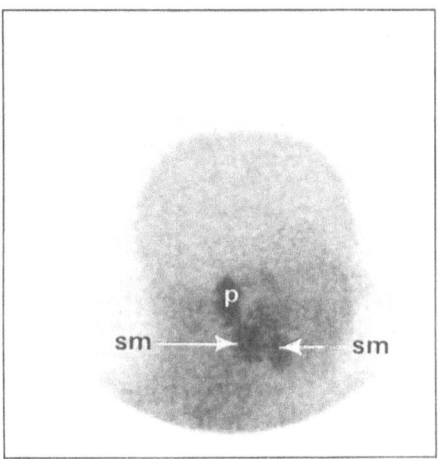

Fig. 4.12.iii. Teenager: right lateral skull

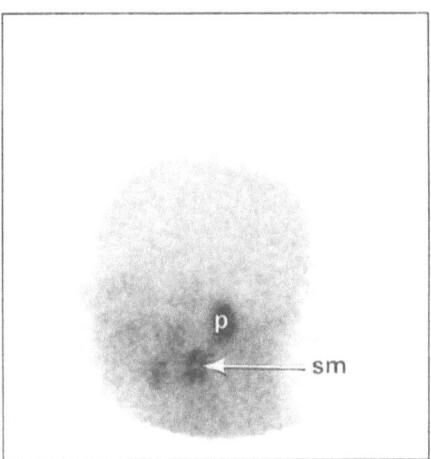

Fig. 4.12.iv. Teenager: left lateral skull

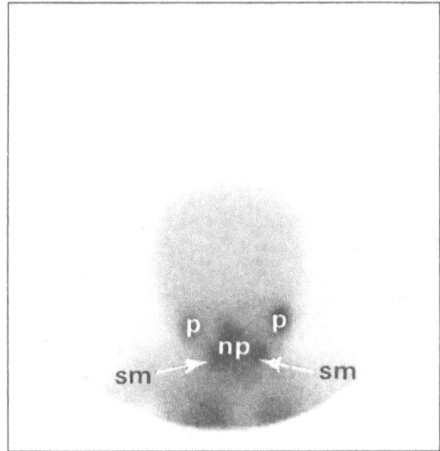

Fig. 4.12.v. Child: anterior skull

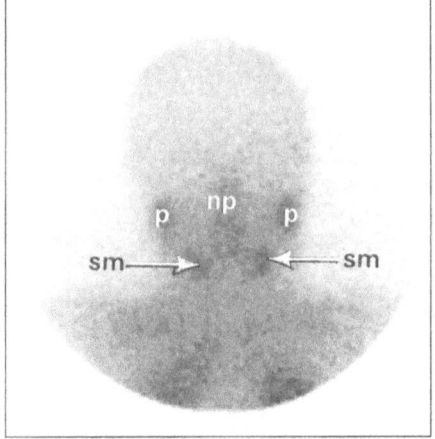

Fig. 4.12.vi. Teenager: anterior skull

Key: *p*, parotid gland; *sm*, submandibular gland; *t*, thyroid; *np*, nasopharynx

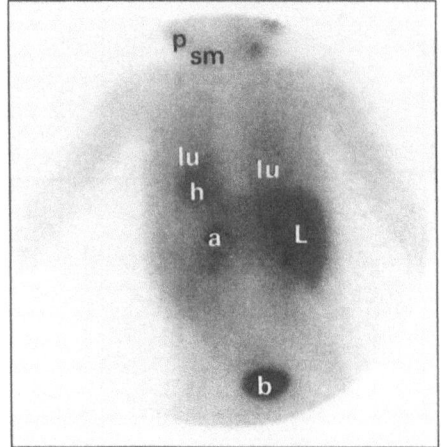

Fig. 4.13.i. Baby: posterior chest and abdomen

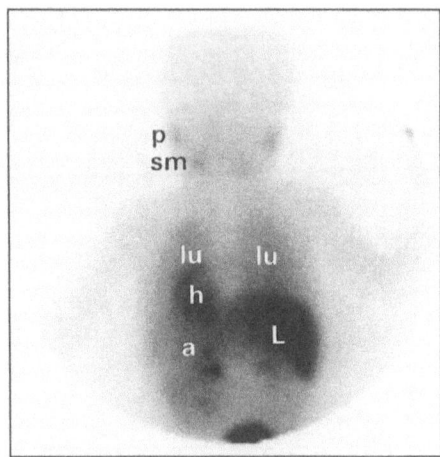

Fig. 4.13.ii. Baby: posterior chest

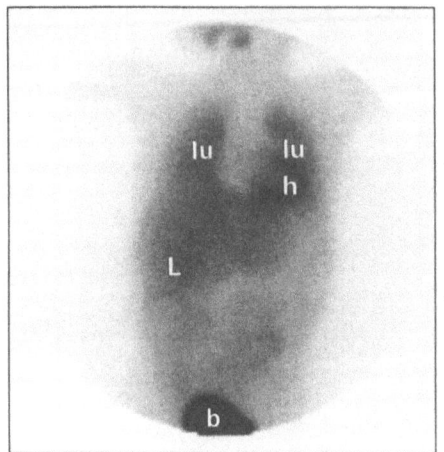

Fig. 4.13.iii. Infant: anterior chest and abdomen

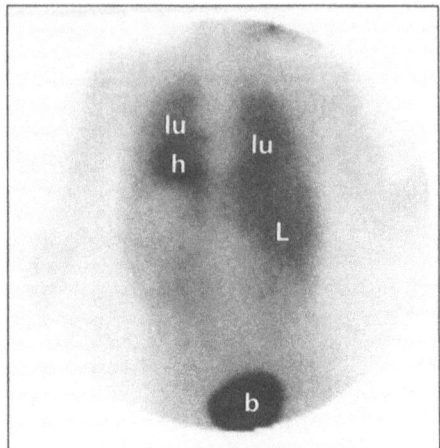

Fig. 4.13.iv. Infant: posterior chest and abdomen

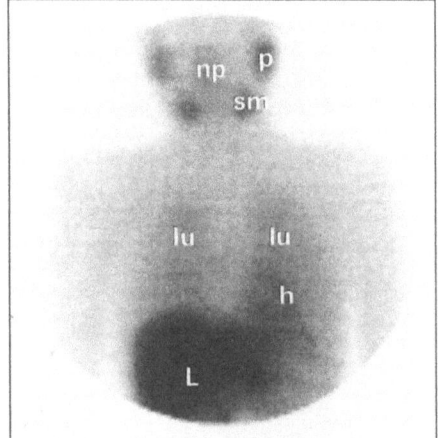

Fig. 4.13.v. Child: anterior chest

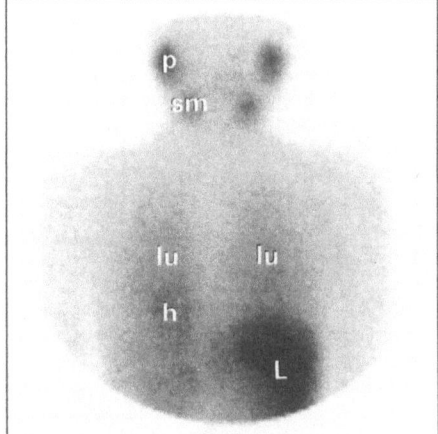

Fig. 4.13.vi. Child: posterior chest

Key: *p*, parotid gland; *sm*, submandibular gland; *np*, nasopharynx; *lu*, lung; *h*, heart; *b*, bladder; *a*, adrenal; *L*, liver

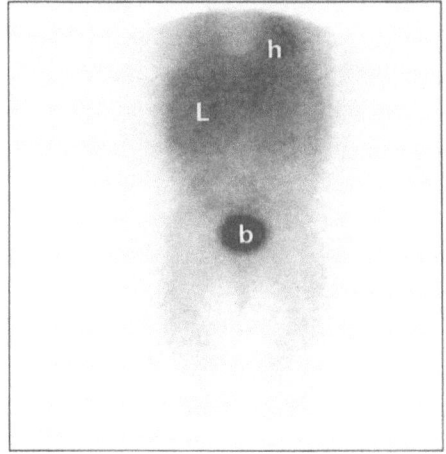

Fig. 4.14.i. Baby: anterior abdomen and pelvis

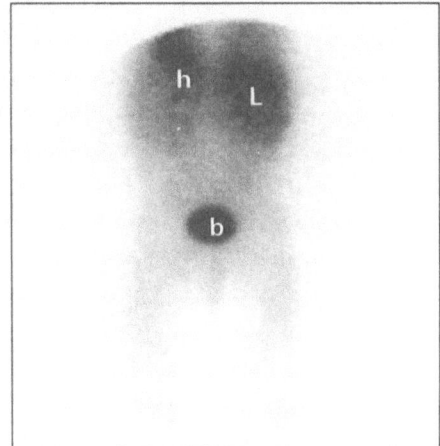

Fig. 4.14.ii: Baby: posterior abdomen and pelvis

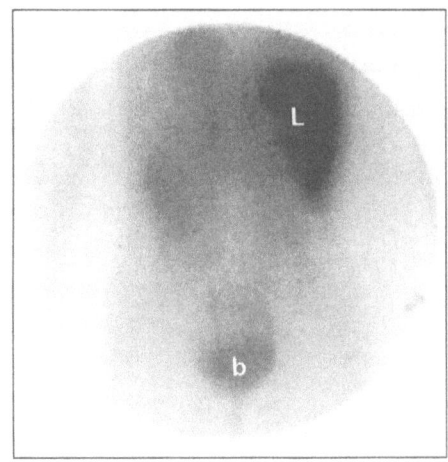

Fig. 4.14.iii. Child. anterior abdomen and pelvis

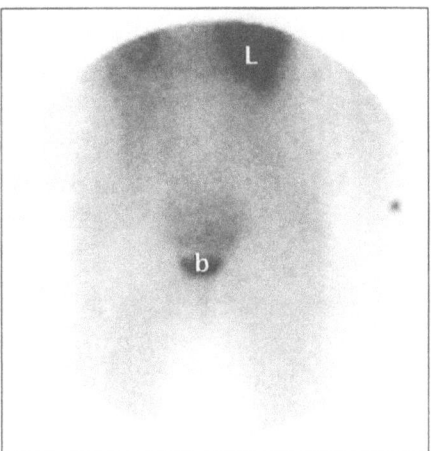

Fig. 4.14.iv. Child: posterior abdomen and pelvis

Key: h, heart; *L*, liver; *b*, bladder

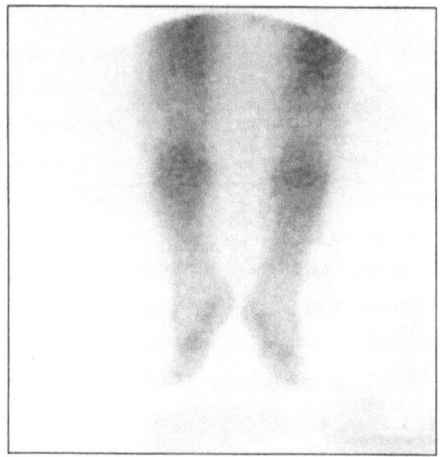

Fig. 4.15.1. Baby: posterior of legs

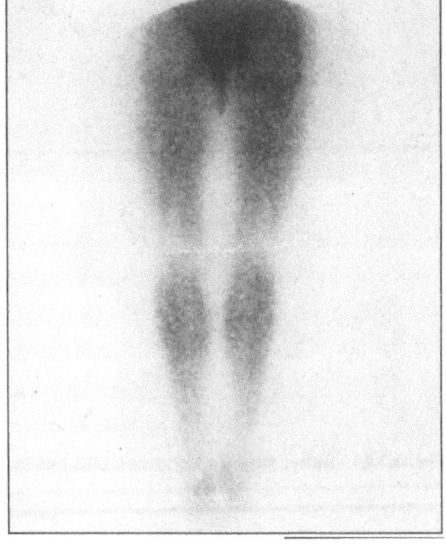

Fig. 4.15.ii. Infant: posterior of legs

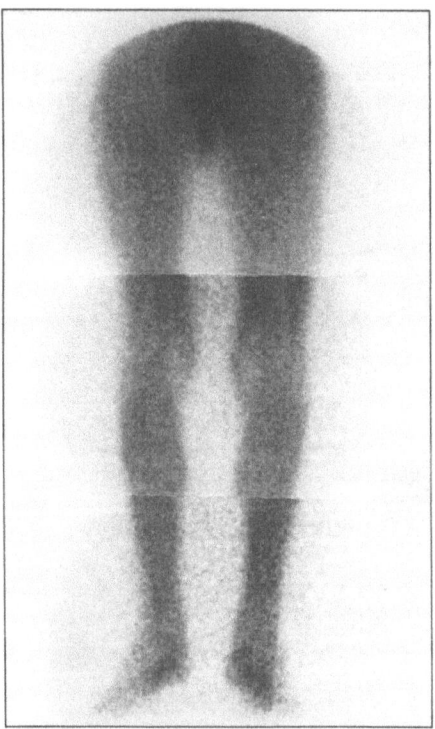

Fig. 4.15.iii. Child: posterior of legs

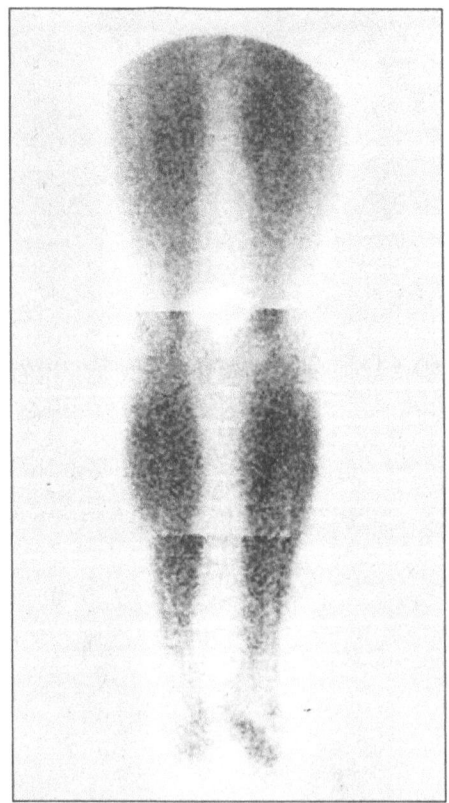

Fig. 4.15.iv. Teenager: posterior of legs

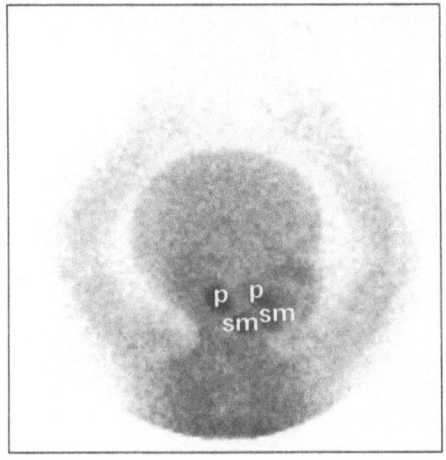

Fig. 4.16.i. Infant: right lateral skull

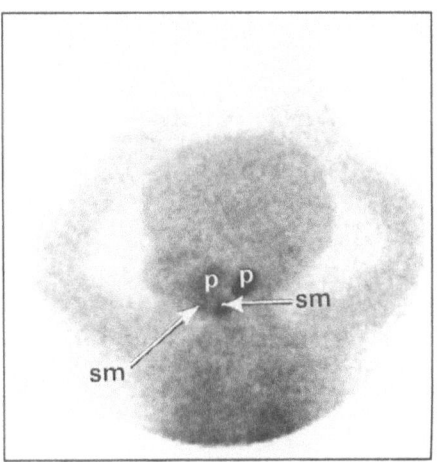

Fig. 4.16.ii. Infant: left lateral skull

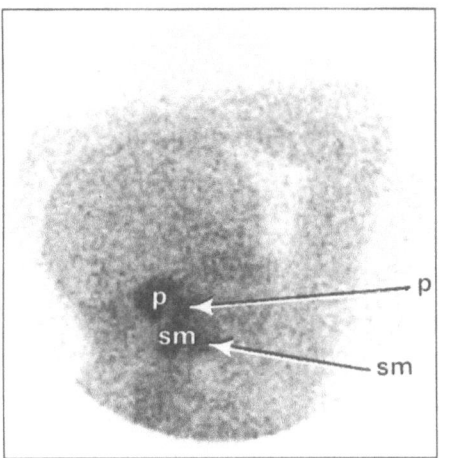

Fig. 4.16.iii. Teenager: right lateral skull

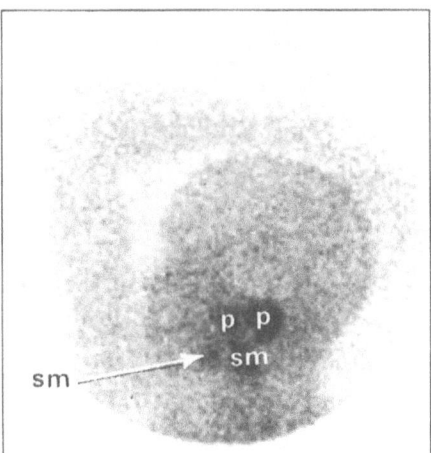

Fig. 4.16.iv. Teenager: left lateral skull

Key: p, parotid gland; *sm*, submandibular gland

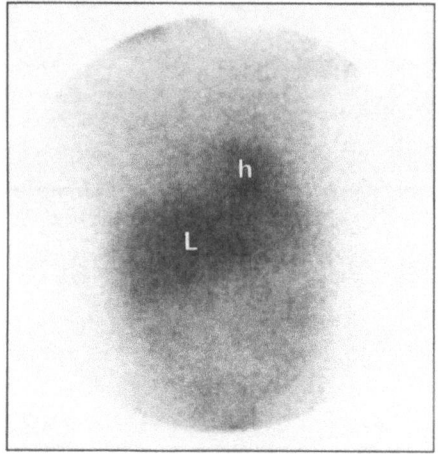

Fig. 4.17.i. Child: anterior chest and abdomen

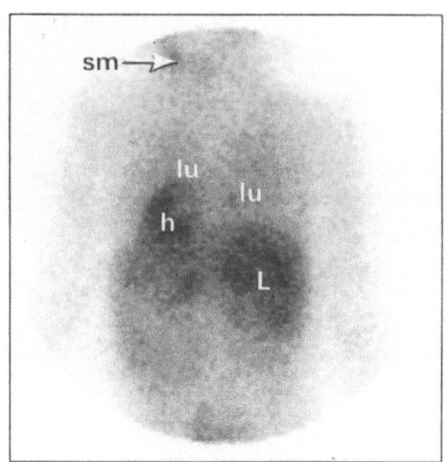

Fig. 4.17.ii. Child: posterior chest and abdomen

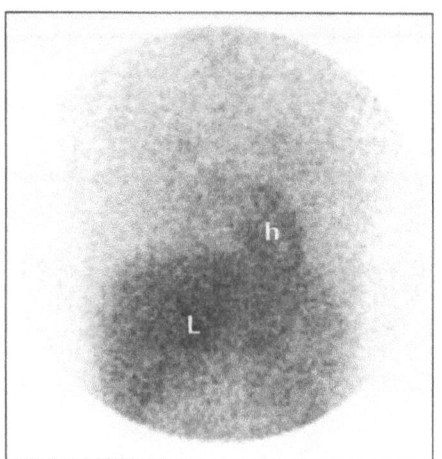

Fig. 4.17.iii. Teenager: anterior chest

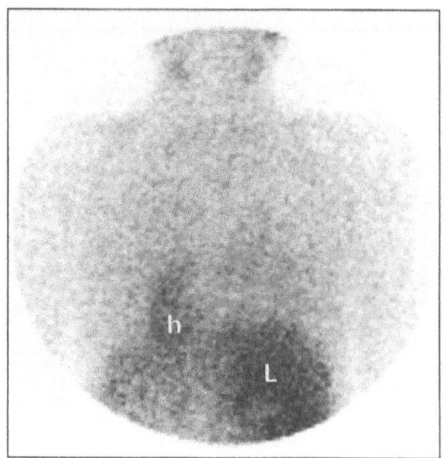

Fig. 4.17.iv. Teenager: posterior chest

Key: h, heart; *lu*, lung; *L*, liver; *sm*, submandibular gland

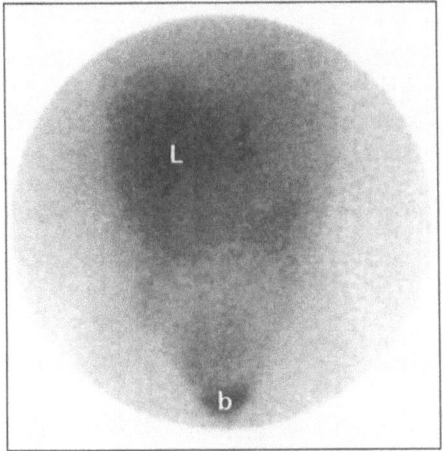

Fig. 4.18.i. Teenager: anterior abdomen and pelvis

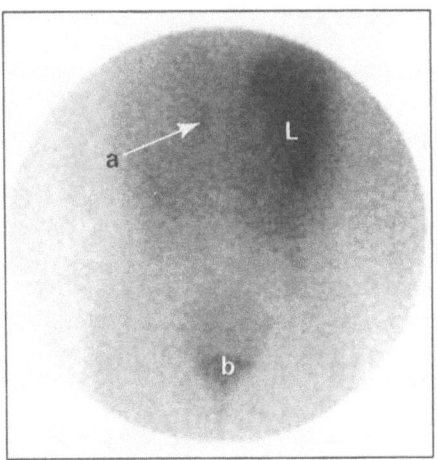

Fig. 4.18.ii. Teenager: posterior abdomen and pelvis

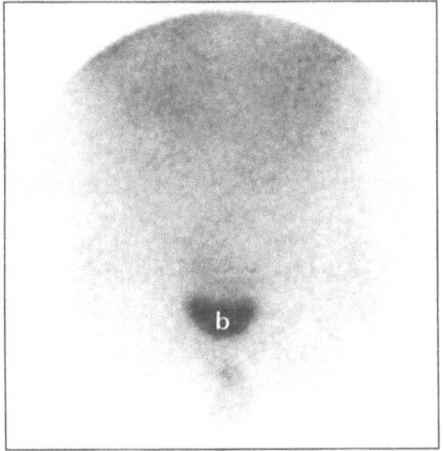

Fig. 4.18.iii. Teenager: anterior abdomen and pelvis

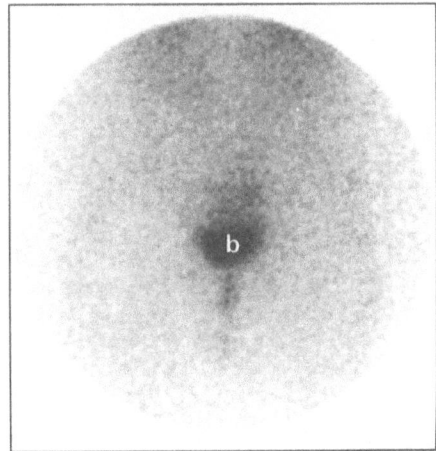

Fig. 4.18.iv. Teenager: posterior abdomen and pelvis

Key: L, liver; *b*, bladder; *a*, adrenal

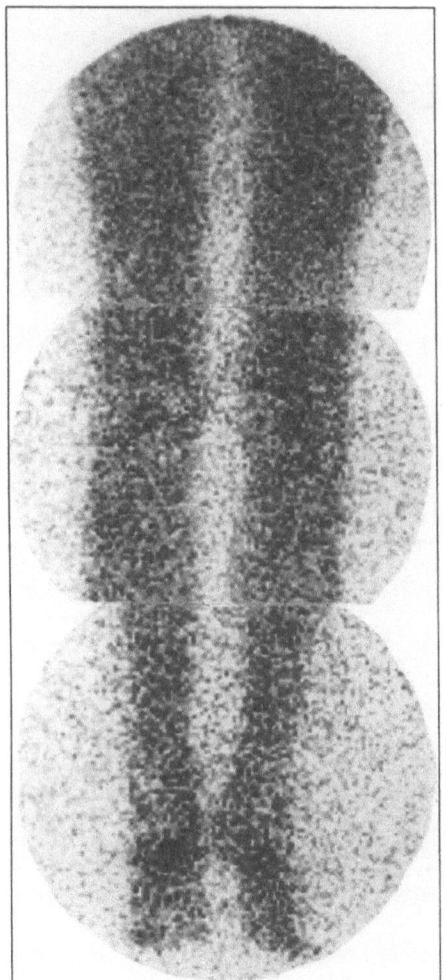

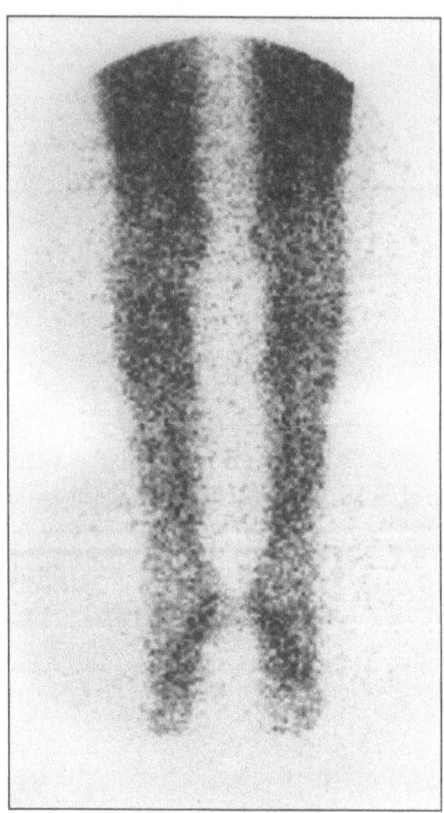

Fig. 4.19.ii. Child: posterior of legs

Fig. 4.19.i. Teenager: posterior of legs

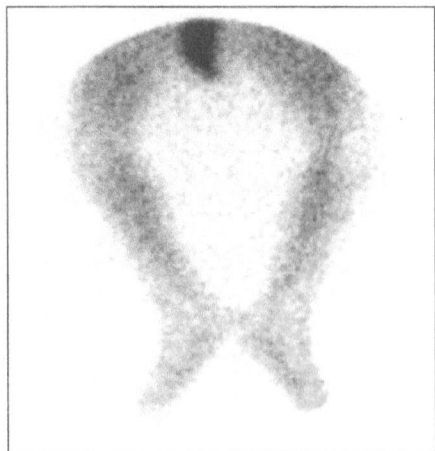

Fig. 4.19.iii. Infant: anterior of legs

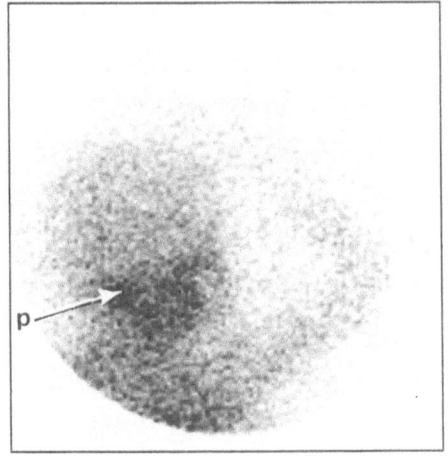

Fig. 4.20.i. Child: right lateral skull

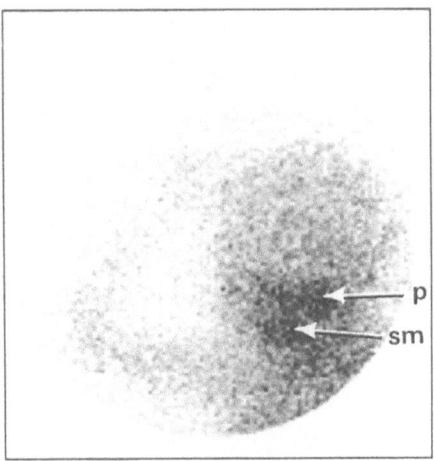

Fig. 4.20.ii. Child: left lateral skull

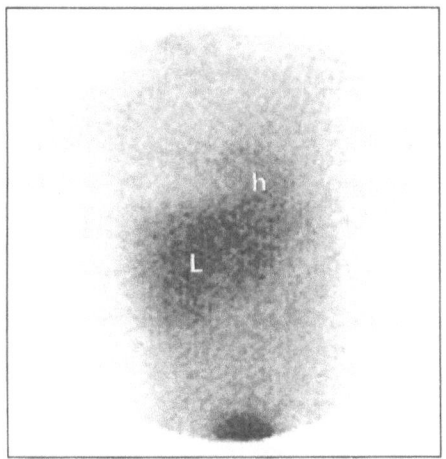

Fig. 4.21.i. Child: anterior chest and abdomen

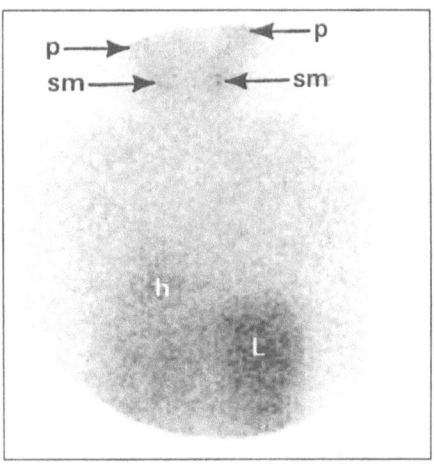

Fig. 4.21.ii. Child: posterior chest and abdomen

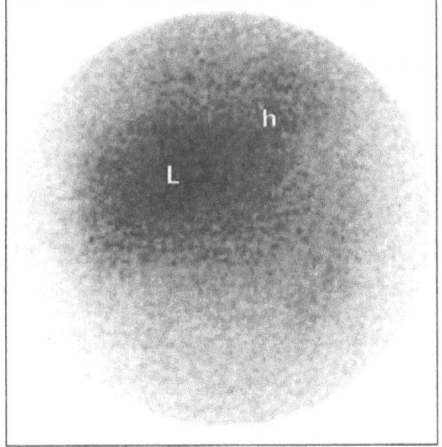

Fig. 4.21.iii. Teenager: anterior chest

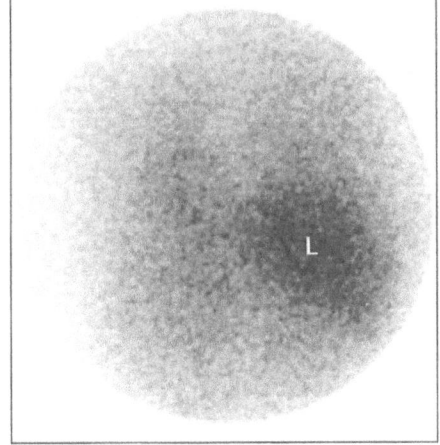

Fig. 4.21.iv. Teenager: posterior chest

Key: p, parotid gland; *sm*, submandibular gland; *h*, heart; *L*, liver

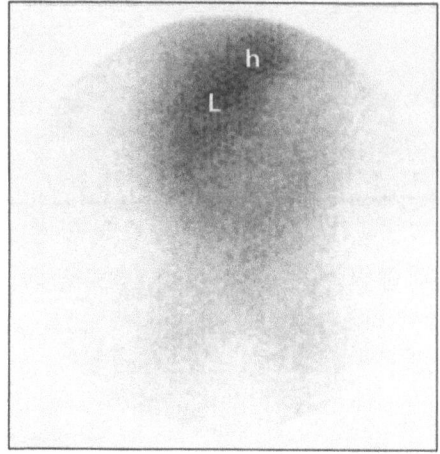

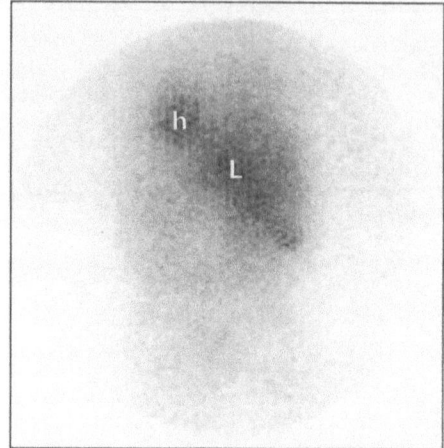

Fig. 4.22.i. Infant: anterior abdomen and pelvis   Fig. 4.22.ii. Infant: posterior abdomen and pelvis

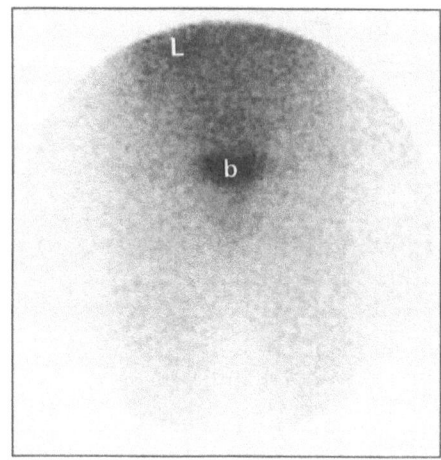

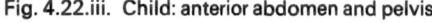

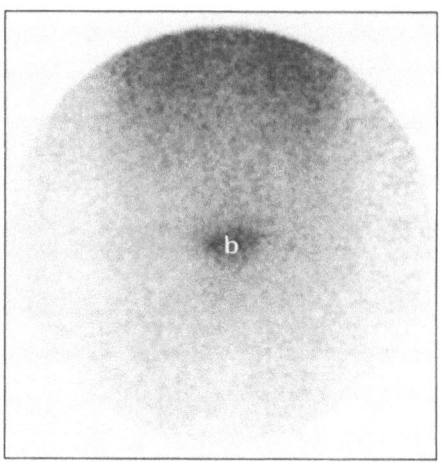

Fig. 4.22.iii. Child: anterior abdomen and pelvis   Fig. 4.22.iv. Child: posterior abdomen and pelvis

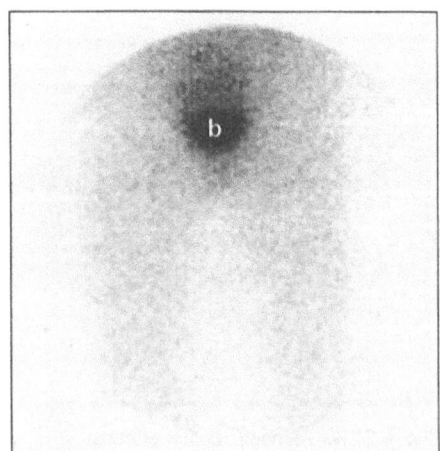

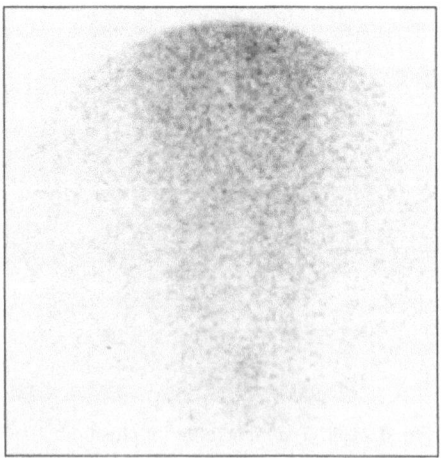

Fig. 4.23.i. Child: anterior of upper legs   Fig. 4.23.ii. Child: anterior of lower legs

Key: h, heart; *L*, liver; *b*, bladder

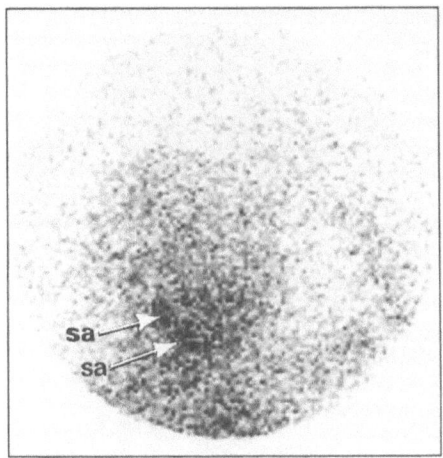

Fig. 4.24.i. Child: right lateral skull

Fig. 4.24.ii. Child: left lateral skull

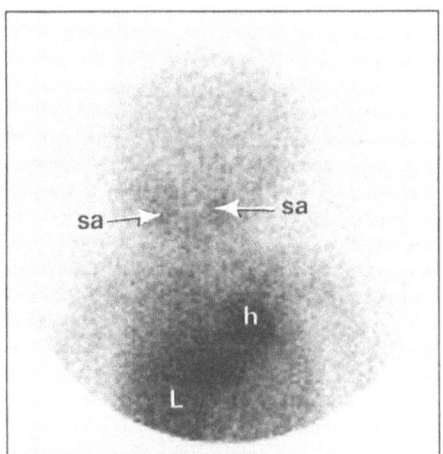

Fig. 4.25.i. Infant: anterior chest

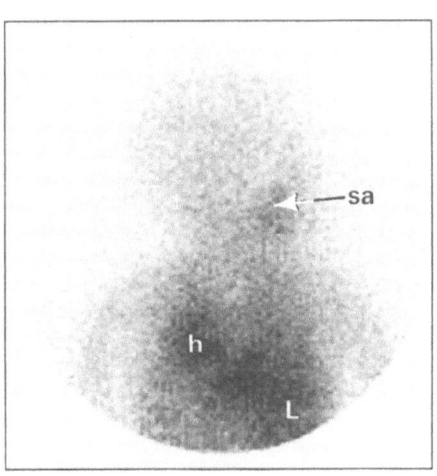

Fig. 4.25.ii. Infant: posterior chest

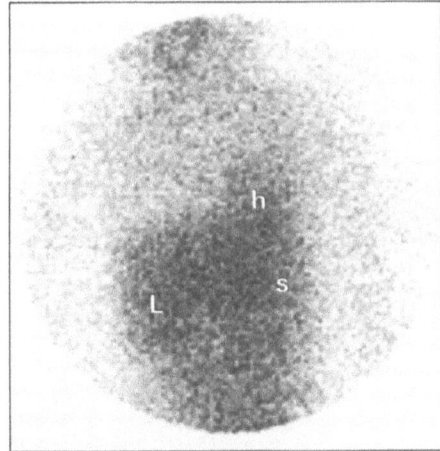

Fig. 4.25.iii. Child: anterior chest

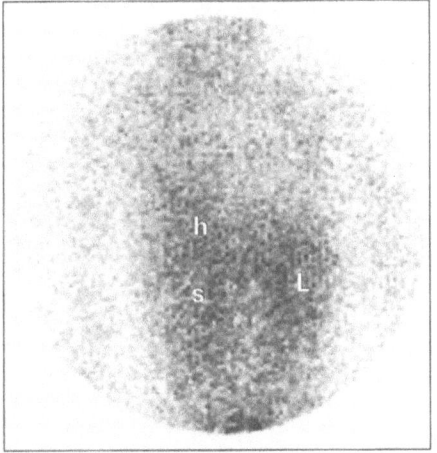

Fig. 4.25.iv. Child: posterior chest

Key: sa, salivary glands; *h*, heart; *L*, liver; *s*, spleen

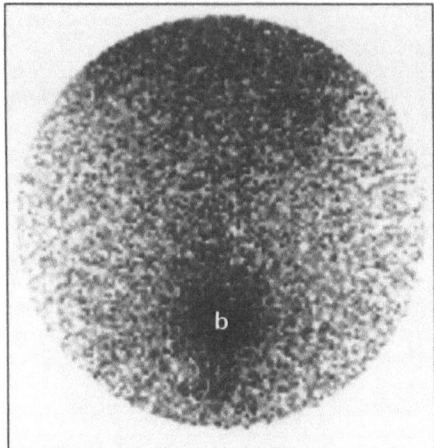
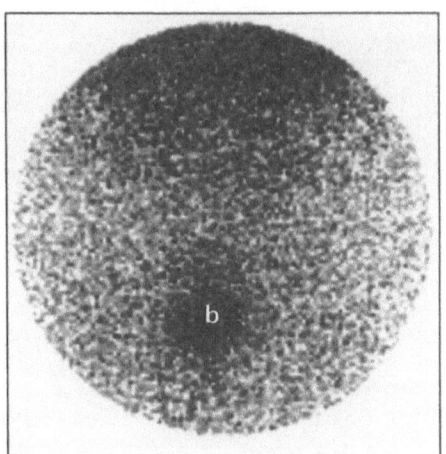

Fig. 4.26.i. Teenager: anterior abdomen and pelvis

Fig. 4.26.ii. Teenager: posterior abdomen and pelvis

Key: *b*, bladder

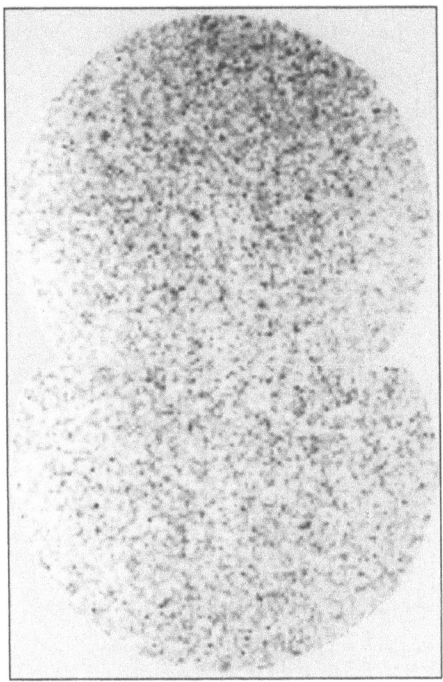

Fig. 4.27.i. Teenager: anterior of legs

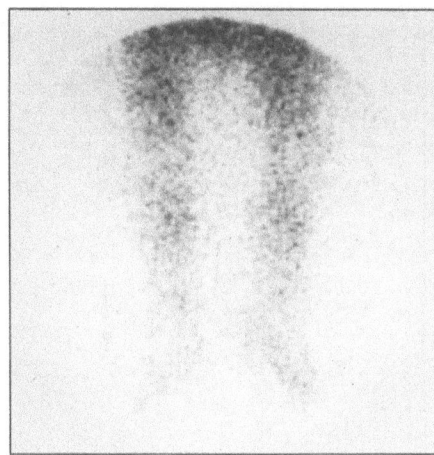

Fig. 4.27.ii. Infant: anterior of legs

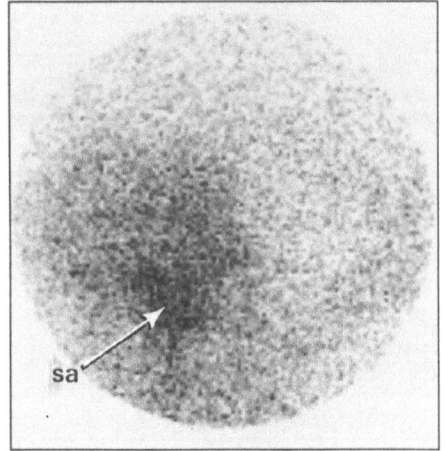

Fig. 4.28.i. Child: right lateral skull

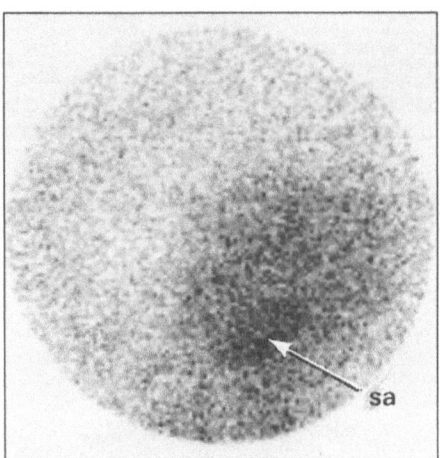

Fig. 4.28.ii. Child: left lateral skull

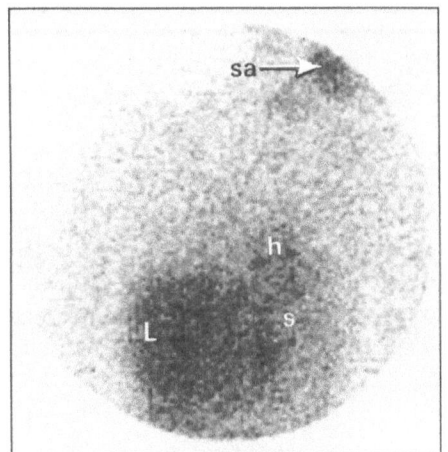

Fig. 4.29.i. Child: anterior chest

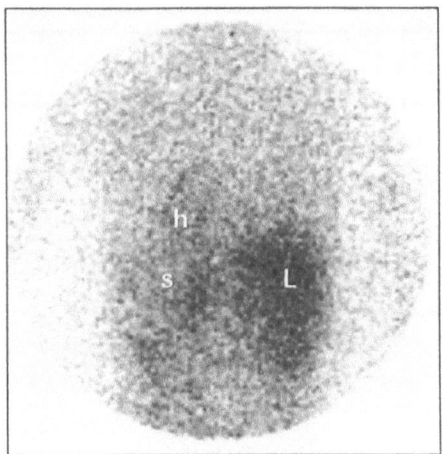

Fig. 4.29.ii. Child: posterior chest

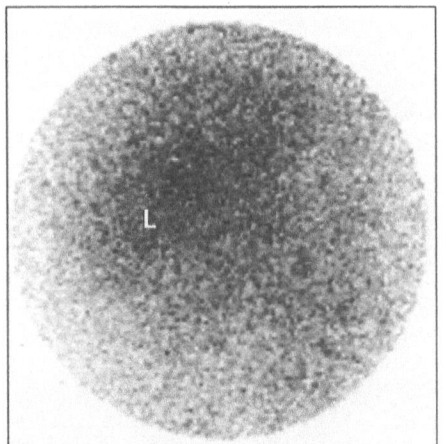

Fig. 4.29.iii. Teenager: anterior chest and abdomen

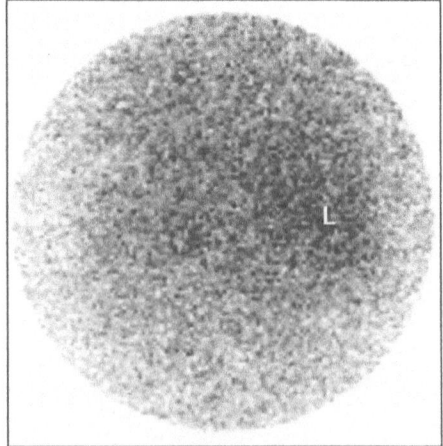

Fig. 4.29.iv. Teenager: posterior chest and abdomen

Key: sa, salivary glands; *h*, heart; *L*, liver; *s*, spleen

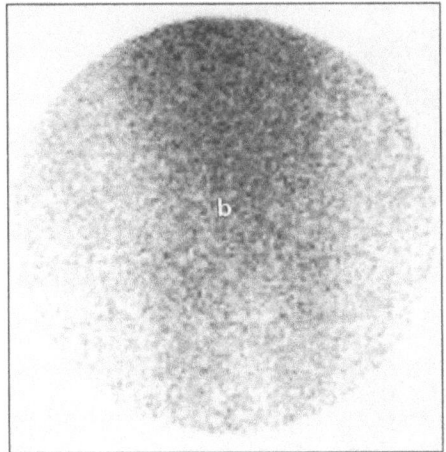

Fig. 4.30.i. Child: anterior abdomen and pelvis

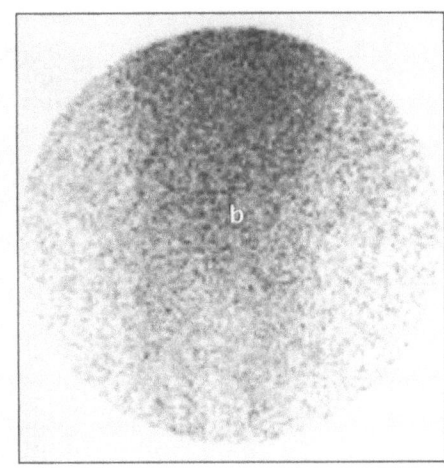

Fig. 4.30.ii. Child: posterior abdomen and pelvis

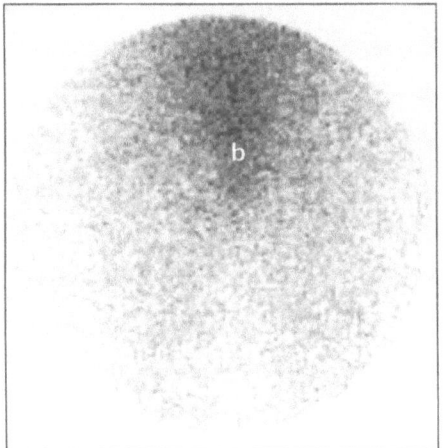

Fig. 4.30.iii. Child: anterior pelvis

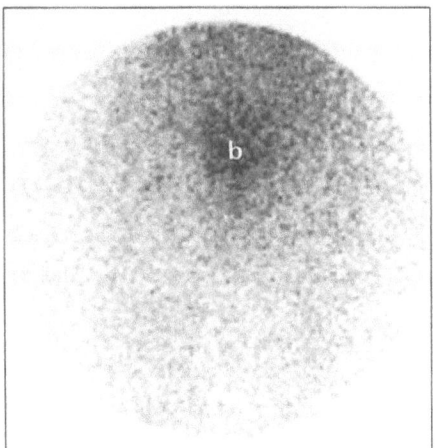

Fig. 4.30.iv. Child: posterior pelvis

Key: b, bladder

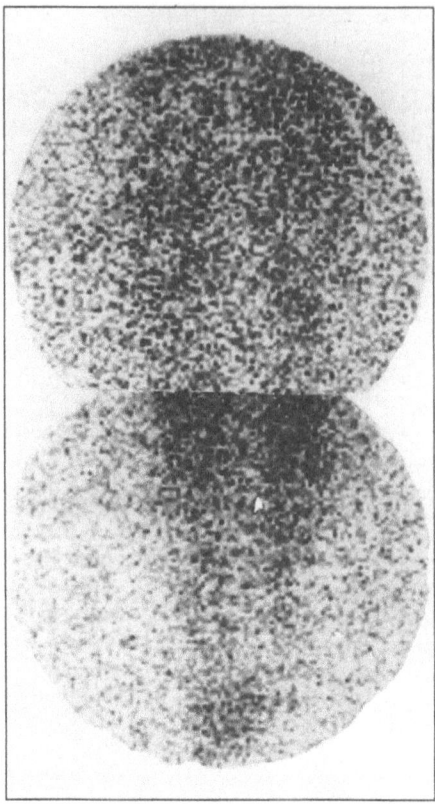

Fig. 4.31. Child: anterior of legs

5 Case Studies with Abnormal Uptake of mIBG

The following case studies have been selected to illustrate the wide range of appearances of abnormal (i.e. pathological) sites of uptake of radiolabelled mIBG in different clinical situations. Each case is an example of either a benign or malignant tumour of the sympathetic nervous system. In some cases the clinical course of the disease in individual patients is followed through, with the appearances of the mIBG studies at diagnosis, remission and relapse being illustrated. The results of other staging investigations performed at the same time are also given. Thus the significance of the result of the mIBG examination may be interpreted in the light of subsequent findings.

Case 1. Stage IV neuroblastoma: right abdominal primary site with multiple bony metastases.

Case 2. Stage IV neuroblastoma: left adrenal gland primary site with a single bony metastasis.

Case 3. Stage IV neuroblastoma: left pelvic primary site with focal bony metastases and bone marrow involvement.

Case 4. Stage IV neuroblastoma: abdominal sympathetic chain primary site with orbital and focal bony metastases, and bone marrow involvement.

Case 5. Stage IV neuroblastoma: left adrenal gland primary site with focal bone and bone marrow metastases.

Case 6. Ganglioneuroblastoma.

Case 7. Stage IV neuroblastoma: bilateral neck disease.

Case 8. Stage IV neuroblastoma: mIBG-negative primary site, with mIBG-positive focal bone and bone marrow metastases.

Case 9. Stage IV neuroblastoma: mIBG-negative primary site, with mIBG-positive focal bone metastases.

Case 10. Stage IVs neuroblastoma: left adrenal gland primary site with liver involvement.

Case 11. Stage IV neuroblastoma: complete remission by all critieria, except mIBG scintigraphy.

Case 12. Stage IV neuroblastoma: complete remission by all criteria, except mIBG scintigraphy.

Case 13. Stage IV neuroblastoma: right adrenal gland primary site with distal lymph node metastases; followed by mIBG-positive relapse.

Case 14. Stage IV neuroblastoma: right adrenal gland primary site with focal bone and bone marrow metastases; followed by mIBG-negative relapse.

Case 15. mIBG-positive ganglioneuroma.

Case 16. mIBG-negative ganglioneuroma.

Case 17. Stage IV neuroblastoma: right adrenal gland primary site with soft-tissue and focal bone metastases, illustrated with planar images and SPECT.

Stage IV Neuroblastoma: right abdominal primary site with multiple bony metastases

History

This 20-month-old female presented in July 1986 with a four-week history of a large right-sided abdominal mass, anorexia, weight loss, irritability, fever, and pain in both legs.

Investigations

A 24-hour urine collection showed raised levels of catecholamines.

An ultrasound and CT scan of the abdomen showed a very large right-sided abdominal mass extending across the midline to the left para-aortic region. Both kidneys were displaced laterally.

Bone marrow aspirates, trephines and immunological marker studies were normal.

The ^{99m}Tc-MDP bone scan was normal.

The ^{123}I-mIBG study (Figs. 5.1.i–ii) showed an area of increased uptake of mIBG in the right and left sides of the abdomen (arrows). There were also areas of increased uptake of mIBG in the left distal femur, and both proximal and distal tibias (Fig. 5.1.iii). There was no uptake of mIBG into the bone marrow.

Comment

The ^{123}I-mIBG study reveals sites of increased uptake of mIBG at points in the long bones of both legs, which coincided with the painful areas found on examination of the patient. These were presumed to be metastatic sites of neuroblastoma. The addition of the mIBG study to the staging investigations resulted in the disease stage being altered from stage III to stage IV with a resultant difference in prognosis. The abdominal sites were more clearly seen on the 4-hour study (Fig. 5.1.i). On the 24-hour study (Fig. 5.1.ii), background activity due to mIBG uptake in the gastrointestinal tract resulted in the right adrenal tumour being less clearly visualised.

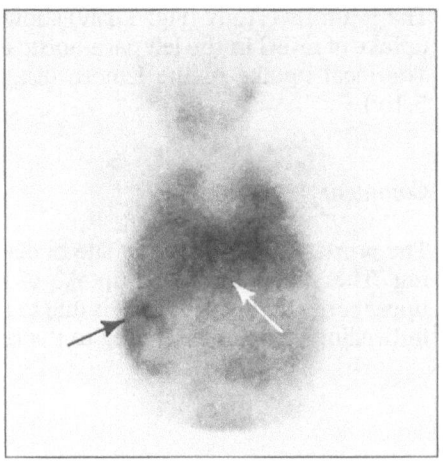

4 hours

Fig. 5.1.i. Anterior chest and abdomen

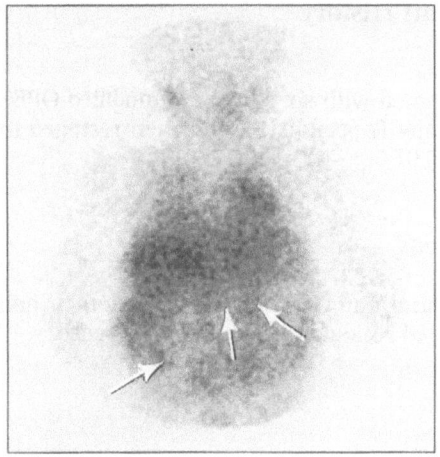

24 hours

Fig. 5.1.ii. Anterior chest and abdomen

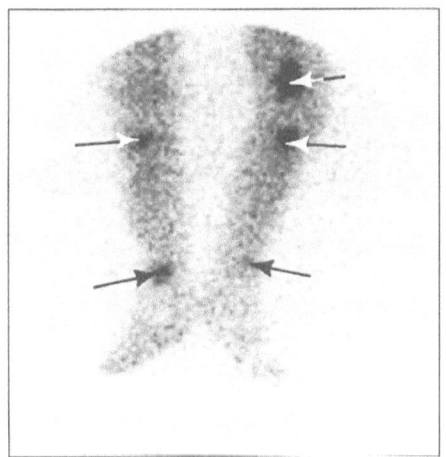

4 hours

Fig. 5.1.iii. Anterior of legs

Isotope	.^{123}I
Activity given	185 MBq
Acquisition time per image	5 minutes
Collimator	low energy

continued

Subsequent History

She was treated with six courses of modified OPEC chemotherapy (Appendix F), and then restaged in November 1986.

Investigations

An ultrasound and CT scans of the abdomen and pelvis showed residual retroperitoneal disease.

The ^{123}I-mIBG study (Fig. 5.1.iv) showed increased uptake of mIBG in the left para-aortic area (arrow). The focal uptake in the femora disappeared (Fig. 5.1.v).

Comment

The primary site is the only site of disease remaining. The site of increased uptake of mIBG in the upper zones of the right lung is due to uptake in the indwelling catheter extending to the right atrium.

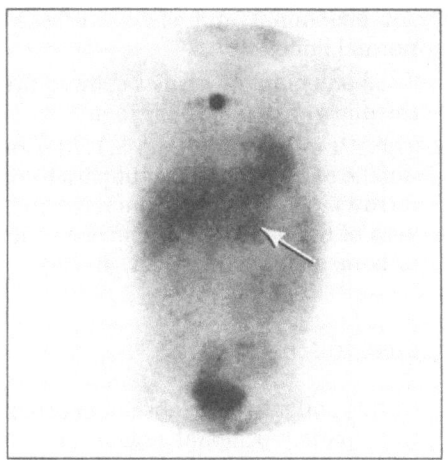

Fig. 5.1.iv. Anterior chest and abdomen

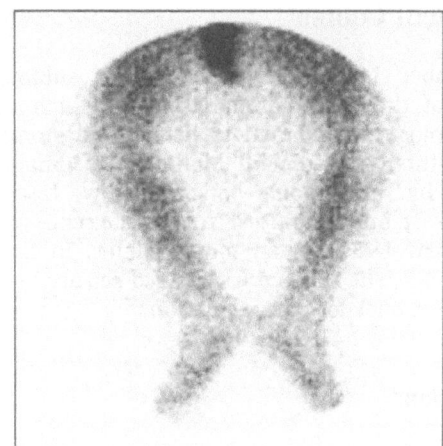

Fig. 5.1.v. Anterior of legs

Isotope	^{123}I
Activity given	185 MBq
Acquisition time per image	10 minutes
Collimator	low energy
Time of scan	24 hours

continued

Subsequent Course

In December 1986, the patient had a subtotal excision of the right adrenal tumour which on histopathology was shown to be neuroblastoma. She was then treated with high-dose melphalan followed by autologous bone marrow rescue (Appendix B), and discharged in complete remission in February 1987. Seven months later, in September 1987, she suffered a left-sided seizure, and was referred back for reinvestigation.

Investigations

A 24-hour urine collection again showed slightly raised levels of catecholamines.

The CT scan of the brain showed a right occipital lesion which on biopsy was shown to be neuroblastoma.

An abdominal and chest CT scan were within normal limits.

The bone marrow studies showed no infiltration of the marrow by neuroblastoma.

The ^{123}I-mIBG study (Fig. 5.1.vi) showed increased uptake of mIBG in the right parieto-occipital region (arrow). There was no increase in uptake in the area of the original tumour or in the cortical bone or bone marrow (Figs. 5.1.vii–viii).

Comment

In this patient the relapse of neuroblastoma in the right parieto-occipital region shows the ability of areas of relapse to take up mIBG. Radiolabelled mIBG does not usually cross the blood–brain barrier; however, in this case neurosurgery has damaged the barrier, allowing passage of mIBG across it and into the tumour.

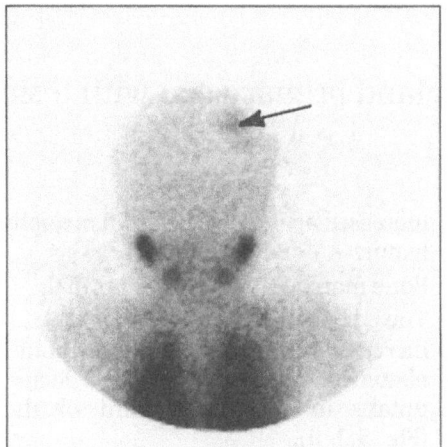

Fig. 5.1.vi. Posterior skull

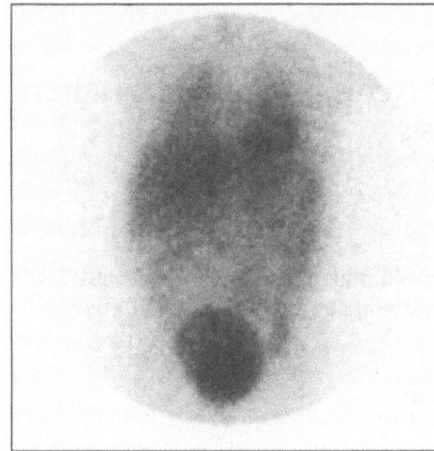

Fig. 5.1.vii. Anterior chest and abdomen

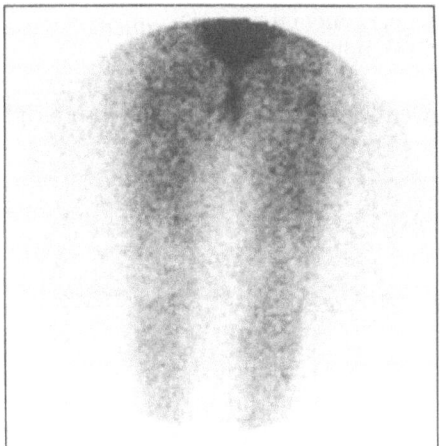

Fig. 5.1.viii. Posterior of legs

Isotope	^{123}I
Activity given	185 MBq
Acquisition time per image	10 minutes
Collimator	low energy
Time of scan	24 hours

Stage IV Neuroblastoma: left adrenal gland primary site with a single bony metastasis

History

This $2\frac{1}{2}$ year-old male presented in June 1987 with an abdominal mass and pain in the left knee.

Investigations

A 24-hour urine collection showed slightly raised levels of catecholamines.

The abdominal ultrasound and abdominal and chest CT scans showed a large retroperitoneal mass arising from the left adrenal, and extending across the midline.

A ^{99m}Tc-MDP bone scan showed an area of increased activity in the distal metaphysis of the left femur.

Bone marrow studies were normal.

The ^{123}I-mIBG study (Figs. 5.2.i–ii) showed increased uptake of mIBG in both sides of the abdomen. There was a single focus of increased uptake in the lower third of the left femur (Fig. 5.2. ii).

Comment

There is increased uptake in the right kidney consistent with a right-sided hydronephrosis.

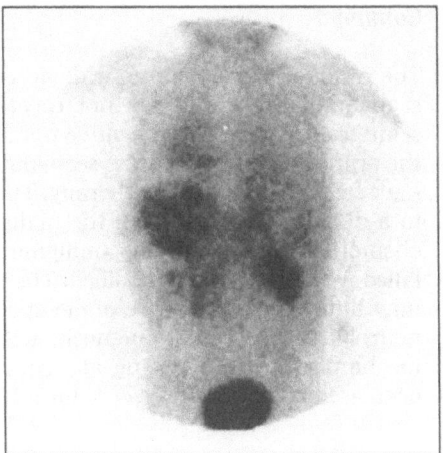

Fig. 5.2.i. Posterior chest and abdomen

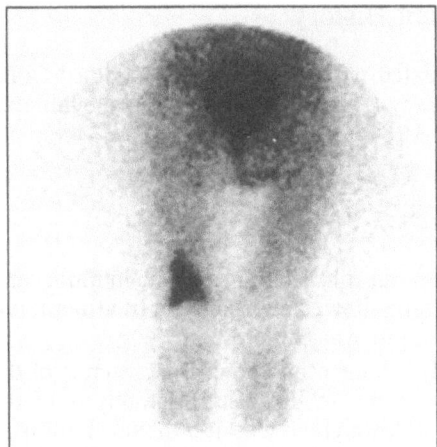

Fig. 5.2.ii. Posterior of legs

Isotope	123I
Activity given	185 MBq
Acquisition time per image	10 minutes
Collimator	low energy
Time of scan	24 hours

continued

Subsequent History

He was treated with six courses of modified OPEC chemotherapy (Appendix F) and then re-evaluated in October 1987.

Investigations

The abdominal ultrasound and abdominal and chest CT scans showed a response to treatment, but residual tumour was still present.

A ^{99m}Tc-MDP bone scan showed persistence of the increased activity in the distal metaphysis of the left femur, although it was less obvious than at diagnosis.

A biopsy was taken from the left femoral metaphysis (the site of increased activity on the ^{99m}Tc-MDP bone scan), and this revealed no evidence of neuro-blastoma.

Bone marrow studies were normal.

The ^{123}I-mIBG study (Figs. 5.2.iii–iv) showed no areas of focal uptake of mIBG.

Comment

The residual primary tumour demonstrated on CT scan and ultrasound was not revealed by mIBG scintigraphy. This false-negative uptake of mIBG at the primary site is sometimes seen after the patients have had extensive chemotherapy. This may be due to a differential response of the malignant cells to chemotherapy, with some malignant cells being killed whilst others are modified. The modified cells may have a different mode of metabolism from the neuroblastoma cells at diagnosis, with the uptake mechanism for mIBG being altered, resulting in a decreased affinity of these cells for mIBG.

Subsequent course

He underwent incomplete excision of the primary site in November 1987, followed by high-dose mel-phalan and autologous bone marrow rescue (Appendix B). He remains in remission.

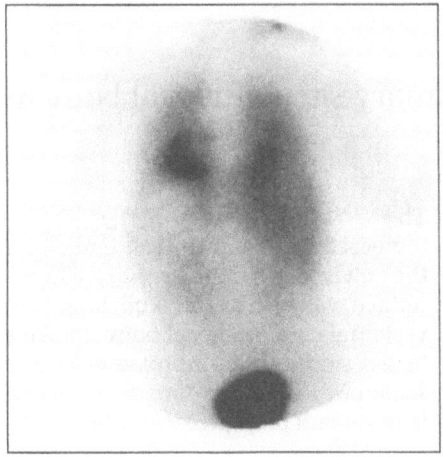

Fig. 5.2.iii. Posterior chest and abdomen

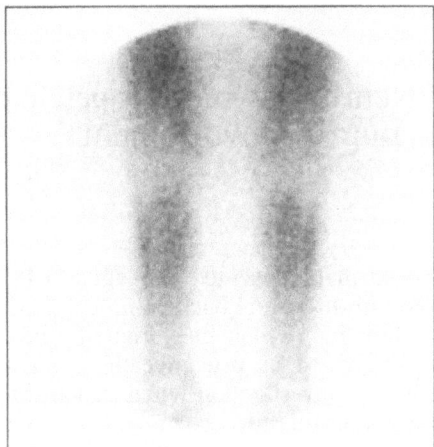

Fig. 5.2.iv. Posterior of legs

Isotope	^{123}I
Activity given	185 MBq
Acquisition time per image	10 minutes
Collimator	low energy
Time of scan	4 hours

Stage IV Neuroblastoma: left pelvic primary site with focal bony metastases and bone marrow involvement

History

This 7½-year-old male presented in August 1987 with a two-month history of back pain, fever, and pain in the right hip, which had originally been diagnosed and treated as osteomyelitis. He was referred for further investigation when he failed to respond to antibiotic therapy.

Investigations

A 24-hour urine collection showed markedly raised levels of catecholamines.

The CT scan and ultrasound of the abdomen and pelvis showed a large left-sided mass posterior to the bladder.

A ^{99m}Tc-MDP bone scan showed increased activity in the right femoral head and neck, and also an area of increased activity in the left hemipelvis.

The bone marrow examination showed infiltration by neuroblastoma.

The ^{123}I-mIBG study (Figs. 5.3.i–iv) showed increased uptake in the soft tissue in the left side of the pelvis (Fig. 5.3.iii, arrow). Diffuse bone marrow uptake was seen in the skull, long bones, pelvis and vertebral column. Focal bony uptake was also seen in the sternum, both proximal humeri (Fig. 5.3.i), scapulas, sacroiliac areas, proximal and distal femora, and both proximal tibias.

Comment

The increased uptake of mIBG into these sites is consistent with a diagnosis of stage IV neuroblastoma, the primary site being in the left pelvis with focal bone metastases and bone marrow involvement. When the mIBG examination was performed the patient was asked to empty his bladder before the pelvis was imaged. It can be seen that had urine been present in the bladder the primary site could easily have been obscured, confirming the importance of obtaining pelvic views with an empty bladder whenever possible.

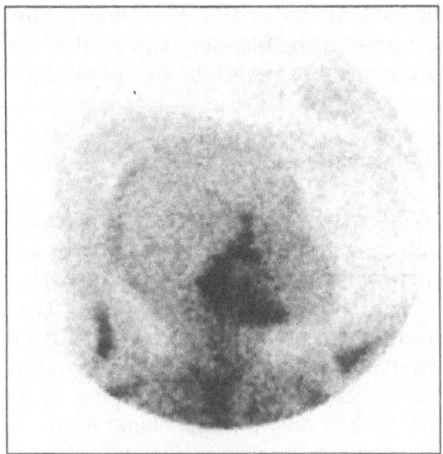

Fig.5.3.i. Right lateral skull

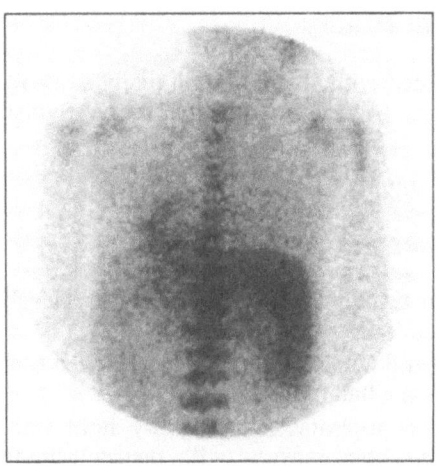

Fig. 5.3.ii. Posterior chest and abdomen

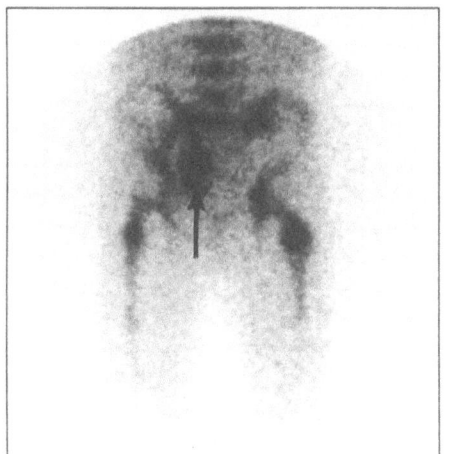

Fig. 5.3.iii. Posterior pelvis

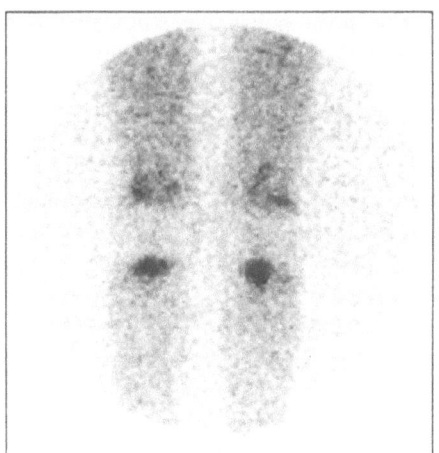

Fig. 5.3.iv. Posterior of legs

Isotope	^{123}I
Activity given	185 MBq
Acquisition time per image	10 minutes
Collimator	low energy
Time of scan	24 hours

continued

Subsequent History

He was treated with six courses of modified OPEC chemotherapy (Appendix F) and was reinvestigated in January 1988.

Investigations

The 24-hour urine collection showed reduced levels of catecholamines.

Ultrasound and CT scans of the pelvis showed that the primary site had reduced in size.

Bone marrow aspirates showed very light infiltration of the bone marrow with neuroblastoma cells.

The ^{123}I-mIBG study (Figs. 5.3.v–viii) showed that the primary site in the pelvis was still visible (Fig. 5.3.vii, arrow), although it was partly obscured by activity in the bladder. The cortical bone and bone marrow appeared to be free of disease.

Comment

A discrepancy exists between the results of the mIBG study, with respect to bone marrow involvement by neuroblastoma, and the microscopic appearances of the bone marrow aspirates. The mIBG scintigrams do not show uptake of mIBG into the bone marrow, resulting in a false-negative assessment. However, of four sites sampled by bone marrow aspiration *only a single clump of tumour cells* could be demonstrated on histopathology. It would be surprising therefore if the mIBG scanning was sensitive enough to identify single clumps of neuroblastoma cells.

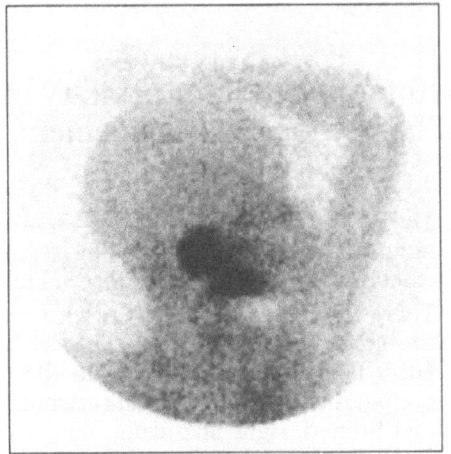

Fig. 5.3.v. Right lateral skull

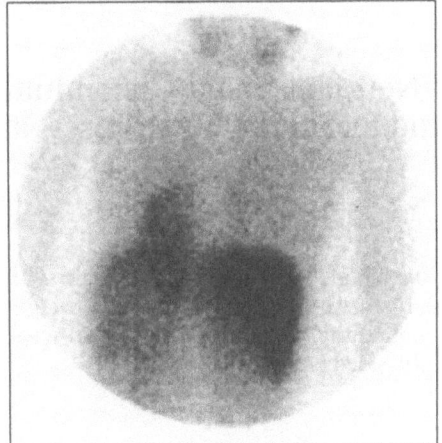

Fig. 5.3.vi. Posterior chest and abdomen

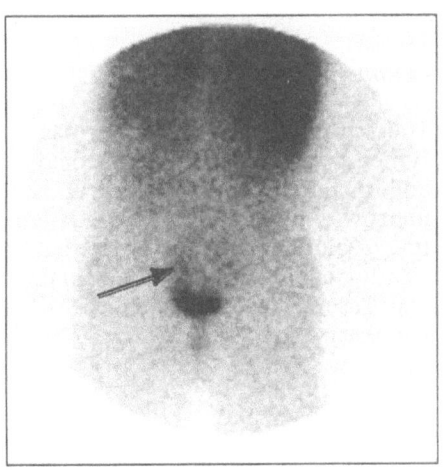

Fig. 5.3.vii. Posterior abdomen and pelvis

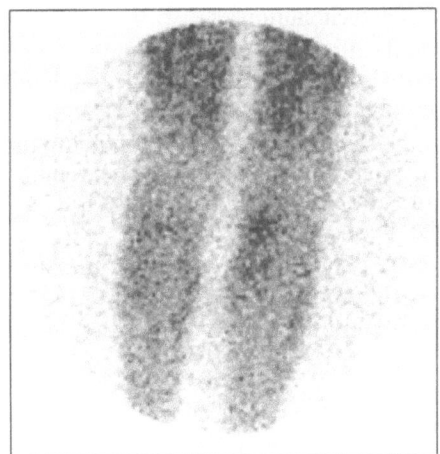

Fig. 5.3.viii. Posterior of legs

Isotope	^{123}I
Activity given	185 MBq
Acquisition time per image	10 minutes
Collimator	low energy
Time of scan	24 hours

Stage IV Neuroblastoma: abdominal sympathetic-chain primary site with orbital and focal bony metastases, and bone marrow involvement

History

This 4-year-old female presented in April 1986 with a two-month history of irritability, anorexia, weight loss, fevers, abdominal distension and a two-week history of right-sided proptosis.

Investigations

The 24-hour urine collection showed markedly raised levels of catecholamines.

The abdominal ultrasound, and abdominal and chest CT scans showed a large right-sided abdominal mass encasing the great vessels.

A CT scan of the brain showed a mass involving the greater wing of sphenoid on the right, extending anteriorly into the orbit, and posteriorly into the middle cranial fossa.

The ^{99m}Tc-MDP bone scan showed increased activity in the right orbit only.

Bone marrow studies showed infiltration with neuroblastoma.

The ^{131}I-mIBG study (Figs 5.4.i–iv) showed increased activity in the lower mid-abdomen extending across to the left (Fig. 5.4.iii, arrow).

There was increased activity in the bone marrow of the skull, long bones and the vertebral column. Focal bony uptake was seen in the skull vertex, occiput, both orbits, thoracic vertebrae, both proximal humeri, right iliac wing, mid-shaft of the left femur, both distal femora, and both proximal tibiae.

Comment

The ^{131}I-mIBG study shows a patient with stage IV neuroblastoma, with an abdominal primary site and metastases in the cortical bone and bone marrow. Although the diagnosis is not in doubt, the resolution obtained with the ^{131}I isotope is clearly not as good as that seen in previous patients (e.g. Case 3, Figs. 5.3i–iv) where ^{123}I-labelled mIBG was used.

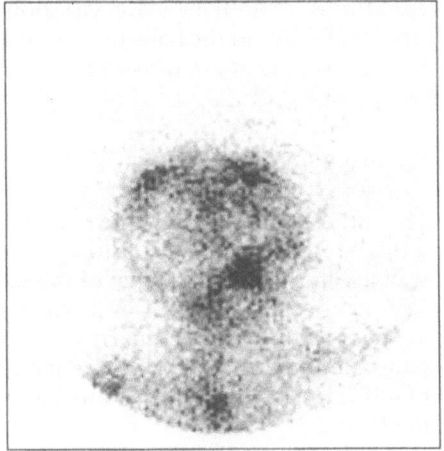

Fig.5.4.i. Right lateral skull

Fig. 5.4.ii. Left lateral skull

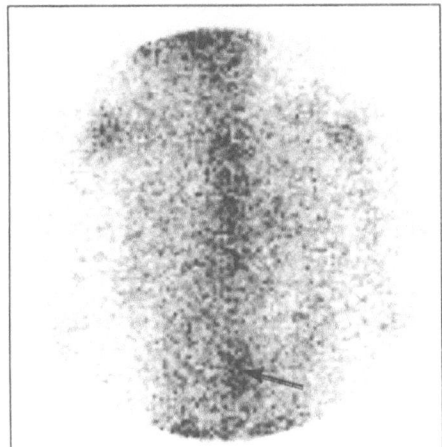

Fig. 5.4.iii. Anterior chest

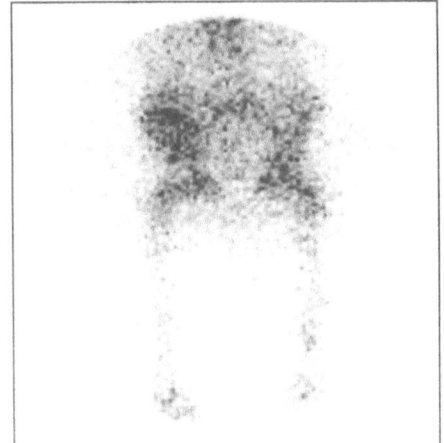

Fig. 5.4.iv. Anterior pelvis

Isotope	131I
Activity given	18 MBq
Acquisition time per image	5 minutes
Collimator	high energy
Time of scan	48 hours

continued

Subsequent History

She was treated with six courses of modified OPEC chemotherapy (Appendix F) and reinvestigated in August 1986.

Investigations

A 24-hour urine collection continued to show raised levels of catecholamines.

Abdominal ultrasound and abdominal and chest CT scans showed a decrease in the size of the abdominal tumour.

Bone marrow studies were negative.

A ^{131}I-mIBG scan (Figs 5.4.v–vii) showed increased uptake of mIBG in the bone marrow of the skull and both proximal femora (arrows).

Comment

The uptake of mIBG within the bone marrow, although present, is difficult to see since ^{131}I-mIBG was used. The bone marrow of the femora can be seen as a central column of increased activity. In patients without bone marrow involvement by neuroblastoma there is a diffuse pattern of uptake of mIBG in the legs, without any specific uptake in the bones.

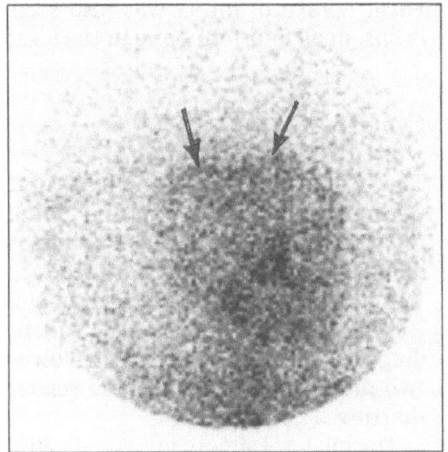

Fig. 5.4.v. Right lateral skull

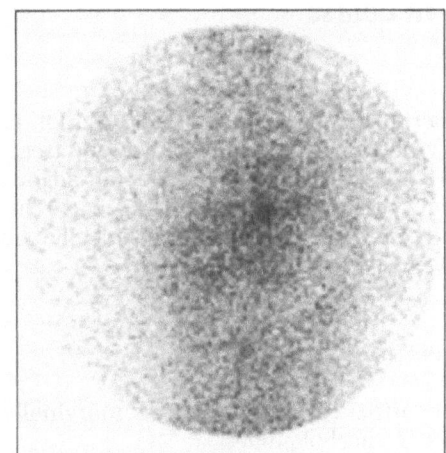

Fig. 5.4.vi. Anterior chest

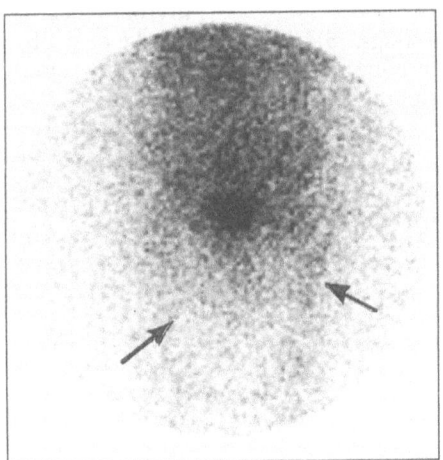

Fig. 5.4.vii. Anterior abdomen and pelvis

Isotope	^{131}I
Activity given	18 MBq
Acquisition time per image	20 minutes
Collimator	high energy
Time of scan	48 hours

continued

Subsequent Course

In September 1986 she had a subtotal excision of the primary abdominal tumour followed by treatment with high-dose melphalan and autologous bone marrow rescue (Appendix B). She was reinvestigated in December 1986 when clinically she was very well.

Investigations

A 24-hour urine collection showed marginally raised levels of catecholamines.

Bone marrow studies were non-diagnostic and showed abnormal, suspicious cells on aspirate, but normal cells on trephine.

^{123}I-mIBG examination showed (Figs. 5.4.viii–x) increased uptake of mIBG in the bone marrow of the skull, long bones and the vertebral column.

Focal uptake of mIBG was also seen behind both orbits, in all four limbs and in the lumbar vertebrae.

Comment

The widespread bone marrow uptake of mIBG (although not confirmed as bone marrow involvement by conventional bone-marrow studies) is difficult to regard as normal, when it is compared with a 24-hour ^{123}I-mIBG scan in a control patient (see Figs. 4.16.i, 4.17.ii and 4.19.ii). It was therefore diagnosed as bone marrow involvement. Within two months she showed florid relapse in her bone marrow.

The bilateral sites of increased activity seen in the skull (Fig. 5.4.ix, arrows) is due to parotid uptake of mIBG. Refusal by the patient to take the prescribed thyroid-blocking medication resulted in intense uptake of ^{123}I by the thyroid (Figs. 5.4.viii–ix). This was only discovered after the examinaton was finished.

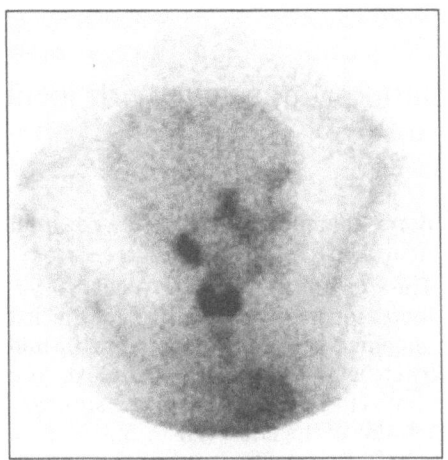

Fig. 5.4.viii. Right lateral skull

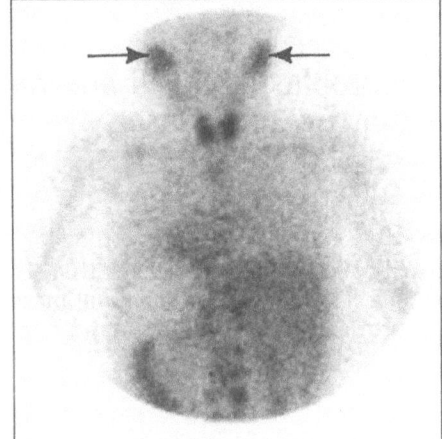

Fig. 5.4.ix. Posterior chest

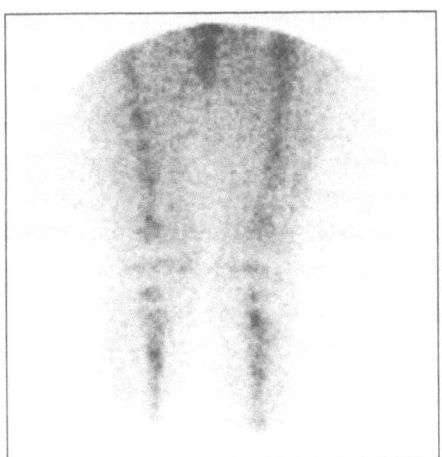

Fig. 5.4.x. Anterior of legs

Isotope	^{123}I
Activity given	185 MBq
Acquisition time per image	10 minutes
Collimator	low energy
Time of scan	24 hours

Stage IV Neuroblastoma: left adrenal gland primary site with focal bone and bone marrow metastases

History

This 2½-year-old male patient presented with a six-week history of a large left-sided abdominal mass, irritability, anorexia, weight loss, fever and bone pain.

Investigations

A 24-hour urine collection showed markedly raised levels of catecholamines.

Abdominal ultrasound and abdominal and chest CT scans showed a large left-sided abdominal mass extending into the posterior mediastinum, and associated with upper right para-aortic lymphadenopathy.

A ^{99m}Tc-MDP bone scan showed no evidence of skeletal metastases.

Bone marrow studies showed infiltration with neuroblastoma.

The ^{123}I-mIBG study (Figs. 5.5.i–v) showed increased uptake of mIBG in the left side of the abdomen with extension across the midline (arrow). There was also increased uptake into a site (presumed to be soft tissue) in the superior aspect of the left side of the chest (Fig. 5.5.ii, arrow). Widespread uptake into the bone marrow was seen in the skull, long bones, vertebral column, pelvis and ribs. Focal bony uptake was seen in the pelvis, proximal and distal femora, and proximal tibiae.

Comment

Once again the mIBG examination shows focal bony sites of disease consistent with the patient's clinical condition, although the bone scintigrams were negative.

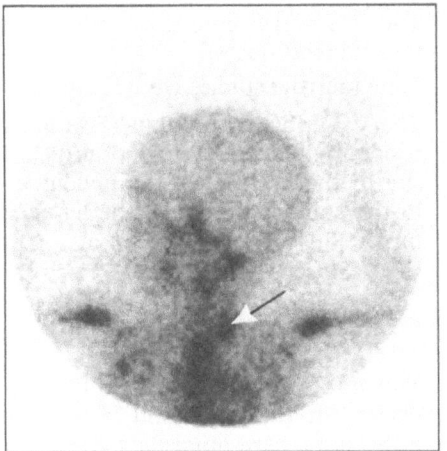

Fig.5.5.i. Left lateral skull

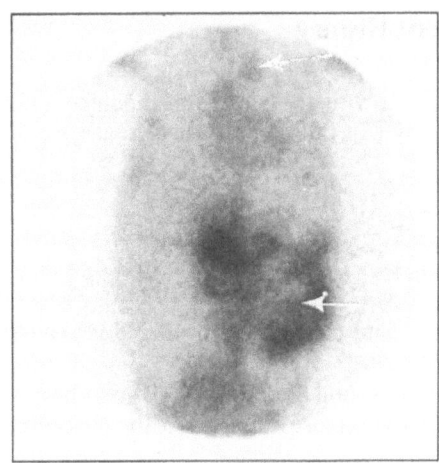

Fig. 5.5.ii. Anterior chest and abdomen

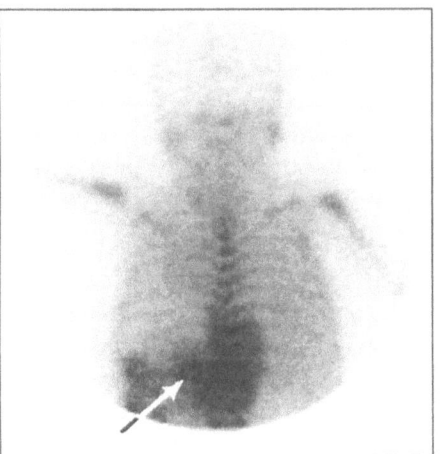

Fig. 5.5.iii. Posterior chest

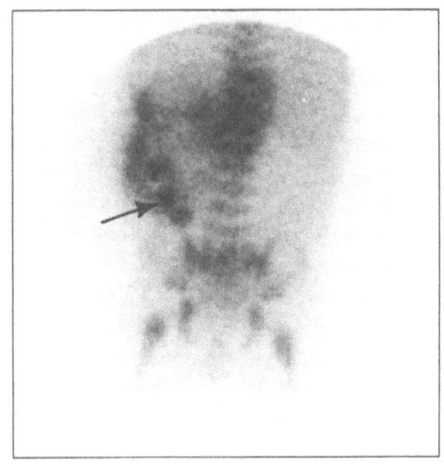

Fig. 5.5.iv. Posterior abdomen and pelvis

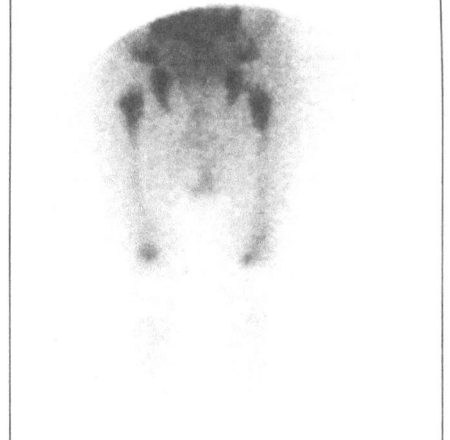

Fig. 5.5.v. Posterior of upper legs

Isotope	^{123}I
Activity given	185 MBq
Acquisition time per image	10 minutes
Collimator	low energy
Time of scan	24 hours

continued

Subsequent History

He was treated with six courses of modified OPEC chemotherapy (Appendix F) and was reassessed in June 1987.

Investigations

The 24-hour urine collection showed reduced levels of catecholamines.

Abdominal ultasound and abdominal and chest CT scans showed a decrease in the size of the abdominal mass.

The ^{99m}Tc-MDP bone scan showed no evidence of skeletal metastases.

Bone marrow studies were normal.

The ^{123}I-mIBG scintigrams (Figs 5.5.vi–ix) showed residual abnormal uptake of mIBG at the primary site in the left side of the abdomen (arrow), and in the superior aspect of the left side of the chest (arrow).

Comment

The mIBG shows clearing of metastatic sites of disease in the bone and bone marrow, leaving mIBG-positive residual disease at the sites described.

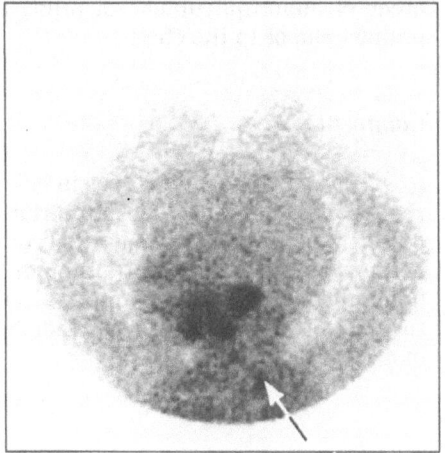

Fig. 5.5.vi. Left lateral skull

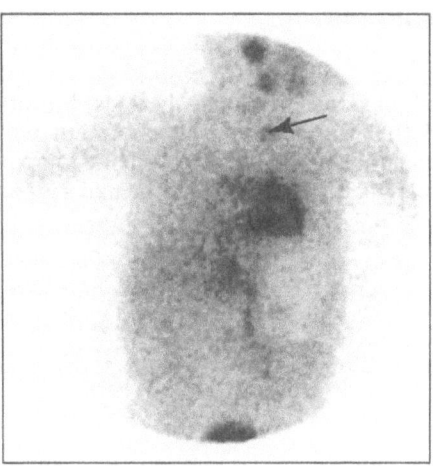

Fig. 5.5.vii. Anterior chest and abdomen

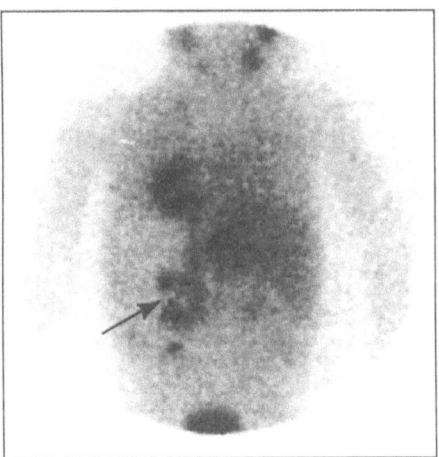

Fig. 5.5.viii. Posterior chest and abdomen

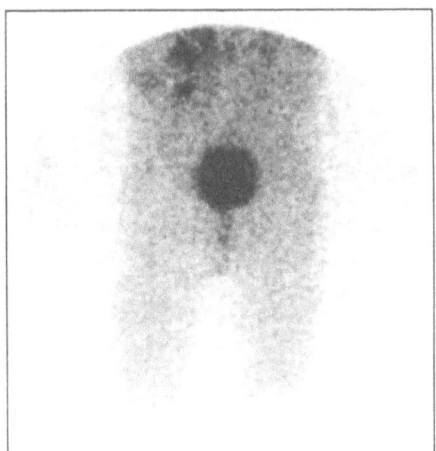

Fig. 5.5.ix. Posterior pelvis

Isotope	^{123}I
Activity given	185 MBq
Acquisition time per image	10 minutes
Collimator	low energy
Time of scan	24 hours

continued

Subsequent Course

The adrenal mass was incompletely excised in July 1987, and this was followed by treatment with high-dose melphalan and autologous bone marrow rescue (Appendix B). Six weeks later he had a repeat ^{123}I-mIBG scan.

Investigations

The ^{123}I-mIBG study (Figs 5.5.x–xiii) showed no areas of abnormal uptake of mIBG at either the primary site or in the chest.

Comment

It was felt that the patient was in complete clinical remission. The indwelling right atrial catheter was outlined by mIBG. Visualisation of the venous access route is a common (although inconsistent) finding when performing mIBG scans. It is not related to the type of catheter, radiolabel or brand of mIBG used.

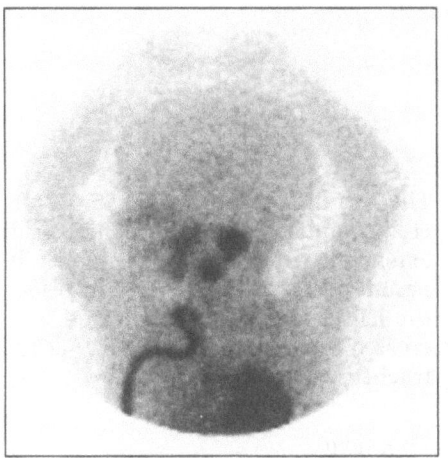

Fig. 5.5.x. Left lateral skull

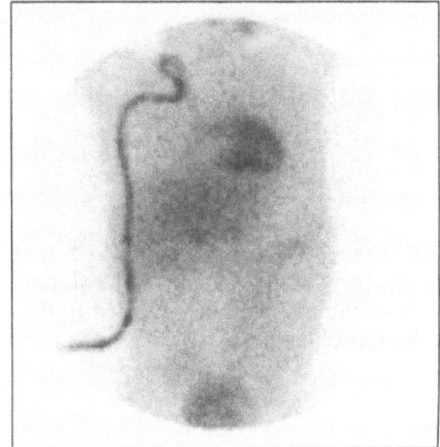

Fig. 5.5.xi. Anterior chest and abdomen

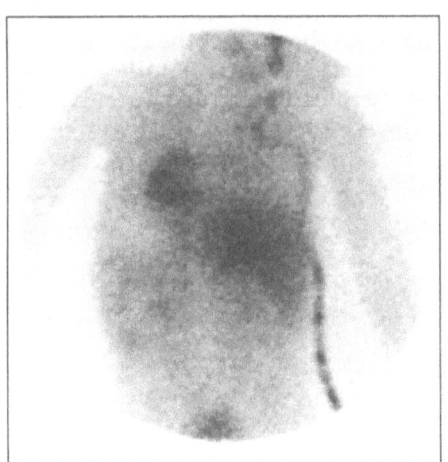
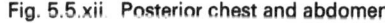

Fig. 5.5.xii. Posterior chest and abdomen

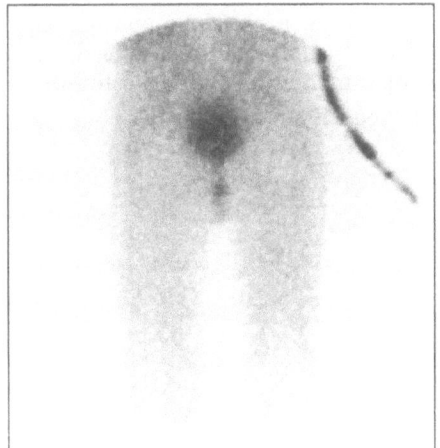

Fig. 5.5.xiii. Posterior pelvis

Isotope	^{123}I
Activity given	185 MBq
Acquisition time per image	10 minutes
Collimator	low energy
Time of scan	24 hours

Ganglioneuroblastoma

History

This 1-year-old male presented in April 1988 with a ten-month history of persistent bilateral neck masses. Biopsy of the masses had revealed a diagnosis of ganglioneuroblastoma.

Investigations

A 24-hour urine collection showed markedly raised levels of catecholamines.

CT scans of the brain, neck, chest and abdomen showed a large, predominantly left-sided, neck mass, extending into the superior mediastinum.

The ^{99m}Tc-MDP bone scan was normal.

The ^{123}I-mIBG study (Figs 5.6.i–iv) showed increased uptake of mIBG into the left side of the neck, extending superiorly to the upper border of the parotid gland and inferiorly to below the level of the left clavicle. The mass extended medially and crossed the midline (Fig. 5.6.iii) at the level of the trachea.

Comment

It is surprising that this well-differentiated ganglioneuroblastoma takes up mIBG so well, since it has been shown that the degree of mIBG uptake by neuroblastomas seems to be directly proportional to the quantity of undifferentiated tissue present (Moyes et al. 1988).

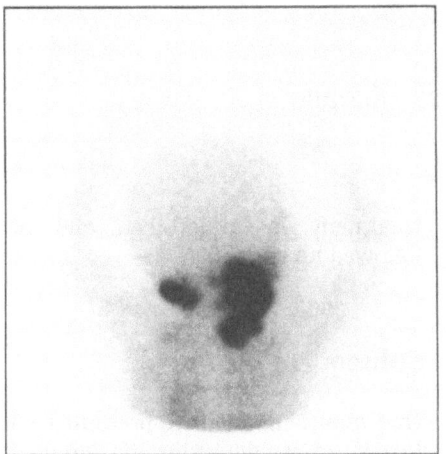

Fig. 5.6.i. Right lateral skull

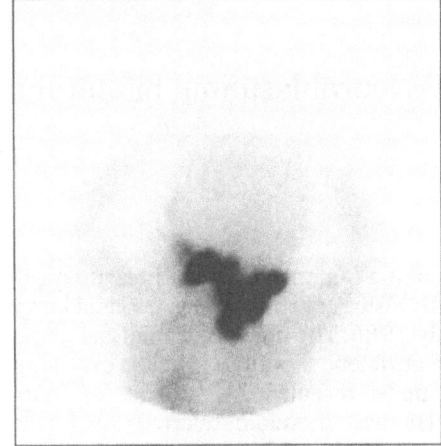

Fig. 5.6.ii. Left lateral skull

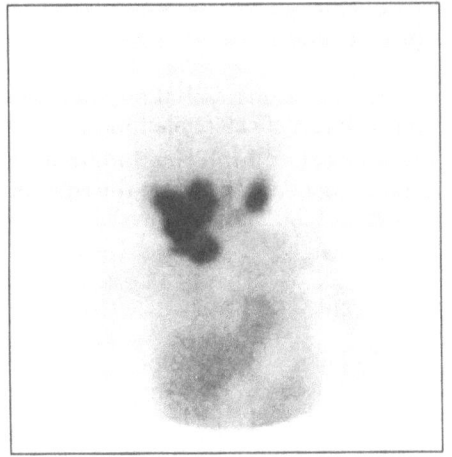

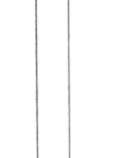

Fig. 5.6.iii. Anterior skull and chest

Isotope	123I
Activity given	185 MBq
Acquisition time per image	10 minutes
Collimator	low energy
Time of scan	24 hours

Stage IV Neuroblastoma: bilateral neck disease

History

This well-looking 6-month-old male presented with a two-month history of enlarged left cervical lymph nodes in July 1986. The nodes had enlarged despite appropriate antibiotic therapy. Complete excision of the lymph nodes revealed the presence of neuroblastoma. He was therefore referred for further investigation in August 1986.

Investigations

A 24-hour urine collection showed increased levels of catecholamines.
Abdominal and chest CT scans were normal.
An abdominal ultrasound was also normal.
The ^{99m}Tc-MDP bone scan was normal.
A ^{123}I-mIBG study (Fig. 5.7.i), showed that the only abnormality was bilateral, symmetrically increased uptake of mIBG in the neck (arrows).

Comment

The uptake of mIBG in the neck was noted but not acted upon since no other staging investigations demonstrated abnormalities in this area. No further treatment was undertaken, and the patient was followed up closely.

Subsequent history

One month later he re-presented with a two-day history of rapidly enlarging lymph nodes in both sides of the neck. He was otherwise well.

Investigations

A 24-hour urine collection again showed slightly raised levels of catecholamines.
The repeat ^{123}I-mIBG scintigrams showed more intense uptake of mIBG in the right and left sides of the neck (Fig. 5.7.ii, arrows).

Comment

Although the distribution of abnormal uptake in the neck is again symmetrical, the intensity on the right side is striking. This was thought to represent neuroblastoma, and therefore he underwent surgical exploration of his neck. Histopathology of the excised tissue revealed recurrent neuroblastoma.

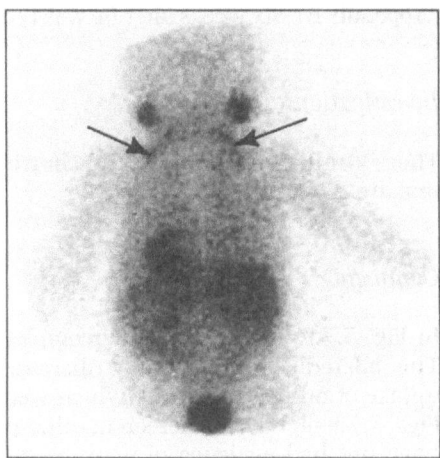

Fig.5.7.i. Posterior chest and abdomen

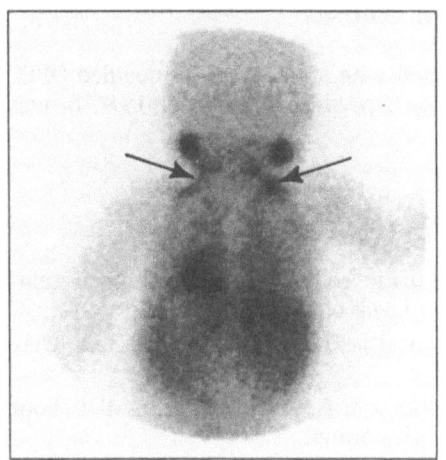

Fig. 5.7.ii. Posterior chest and abdomen, one month later

Isotope	^{123}I
Activity given	75 MBq
Acquisition time per image	5 minutes
Collimator	low energy
Time of scan	24 hours

continued

Subsequent Courses

He was treated with six courses of modified OPEC chemotherapy (Appendix F). In March 1987 he was restaged.

Investigations

A 24-hour urine collection again showed marginally raised levels of catecholamines.
The neck, chest and abdominal CT scans were normal.
The abdominal ultrasound and ^{99m}Tc-MDP bone scan were both normal.
The ^{123}I-mIBG study (Fig. 5.7.iii) showed persistent increased uptake of mIBG in both sides of the neck (arrows).

Subsequent Course (later)

In May 1987 he was treated with high-dose melphalan and autologous bone marrow rescue (Appendix B). Six weeks later he was reinvestigated.

Investigations

The ^{123}I-mIBG scan (Fig. 5.7.iv) showed no abnormal areas of mIBG uptake.

Comment

In Fig. 5.7.iv the neck is now completely normal. The bilateral, symmetrically increased areas of uptake of mIBG in the neck which were present in Figs. 5.7.i–iii, have been seen in other patients who have not had evidence of neuroblastoma. In this child the excision and histopatholgy of one of these areas proved that the areas were in fact sites of neuroblastoma. The decrease in mIBG uptake after further treatment (high-dose melphalan and autologous bone marrow rescue) is consistent with the clinical course. The series of mIBG scintigrams in this patient proved to be very valuable since no other radiological technique provided evidence for the presence of the tumour.

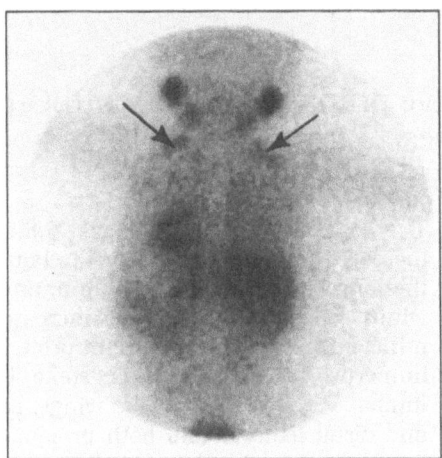

Fig. 5.7.iii. Posterior chest and abdomen

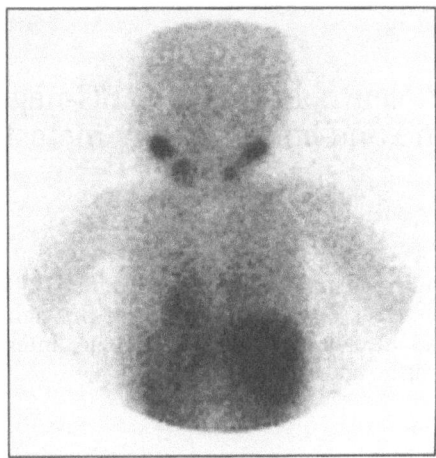

Fig. 5.7.iv. Posterior chest and abdomen, three months later

Isotope	^{123}I
Activity given	75 MBq
Acquisition time per image	10 minutes
Collimator	low energy
Time of scan	24 hours

Stage IV Neuroblastoma: mIBG-negative primary site with mIBG-positive focal bone and bone marrow metastases

History

This 22-month-old male presented in August 1987 with a three-week history of swelling of the right eye. He had also been irritable, anorexic, intermittently febrile, and refusing to walk.

Investigations

A 24-hour urine collection showed raised levels of catecholamines.

Abdominal ultrasound, and abdominal and chest CT scans showed a large heterogeneous mass arising from the left adrenal gland.

The CT scan of the brain showed a large soft-tissue mass in the posterior aspect of the right orbit with no intracranial extension.

A ^{99m}Tc-MDP bone scan showed increased activity in the right sphenoidal bone only.

Bone marrow studies showed infiltration with neuroblastoma.

The ^{123}I-mIBG study (Figs. 5.8.i–v) showed increased uptake of mIBG in the bone marrow of the long bones, vertebral column, and both pelvic wings. There was also focal increased uptake of mIBG in the skeleton: the right orbit, left proximal humerus, left distal radius, some thoracic and lumbar vertebrae, both iliac wings, both proximal and distal femora, and both proximal tibias. The primary site in the abdomen did not take up mIBG, and in fact produced a photon-deficient image (Fig. 5.8.iii).

Comment

This pattern of uptake of mIBG is compatible with metastatic disease in cortical bone and bone marrow. However, this is a very unusual situation where the site of the primary tumour does not take up mIBG, but the secondary sites have retained the ability to take up the radiopharmaceutical.

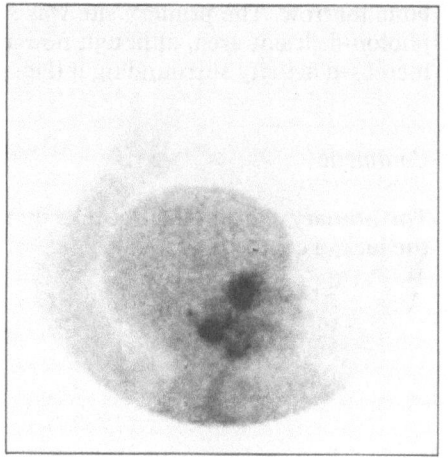

Fig.5.8.i. Right lateral skull

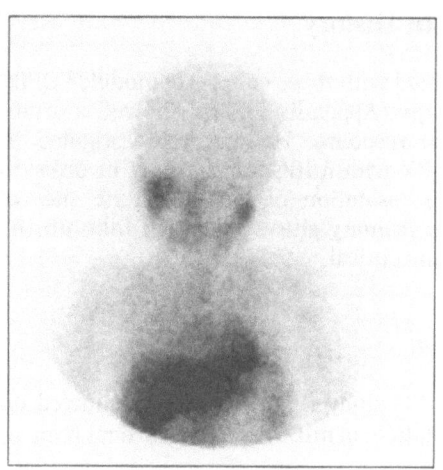

Fig. 5.8.ii. Anterior skull and chest

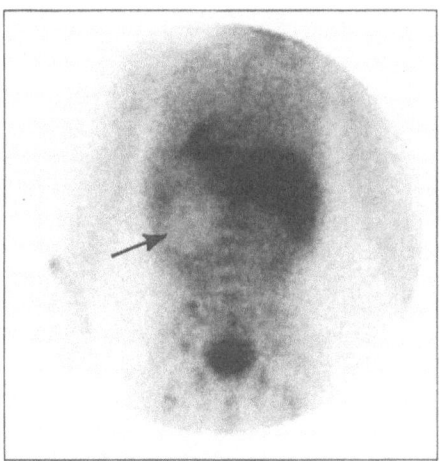

Fig. 5.8.iii. Posterior chest and abdomen

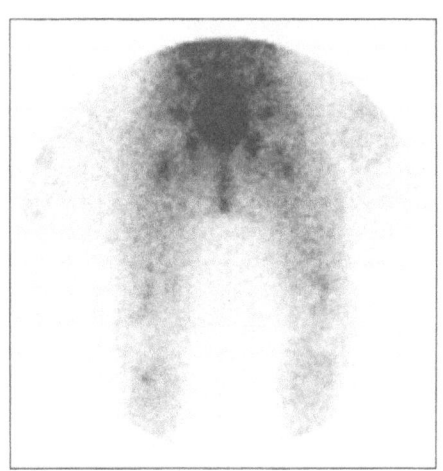

Fig. 5.8.iv. Posterior pelvis

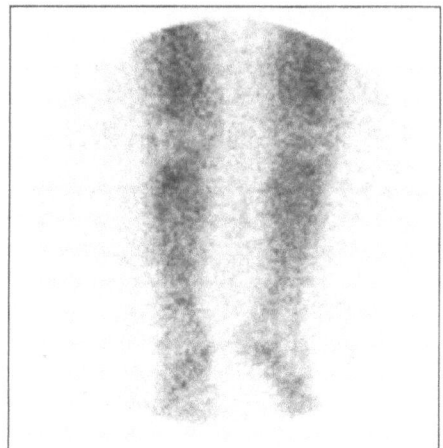

Fig. 5.8.v. Posterior of lower legs

Isotope	[123]I
Activity given	185 MBq
Acquisition time per image	10 minutes
Collimator	low energy
Time of scan	24 hours

continued

Subsequent History

He was treated with three courses of modified OPEC chemotherapy (Appendix F), and showed a dramatic clinical response. He was reinvestigated in October 1987 with mIBG scintigraphy in order to see if, with resolution of the metastatic sites of disease, the primary site would then take up the radiopharmaceutical.

Investigation

The ^{123}I-mIBG study (Figs. 5.8.vi–viii) showed no abnormal uptake of mIBG either in cortical bone or bone marrow. The primary site was still seen as a photon-deficient area, although now with a rim of increased activity surrounding it (Fig. 5.8.vii).

Comment

The primary site still did not take up mIBG despite the lack of competitive uptake.

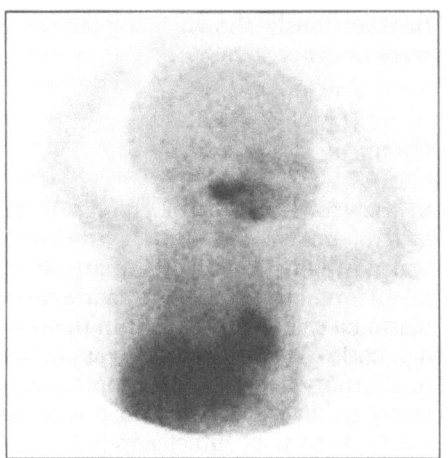

Fig. 5.8.vi. Right lateral skull

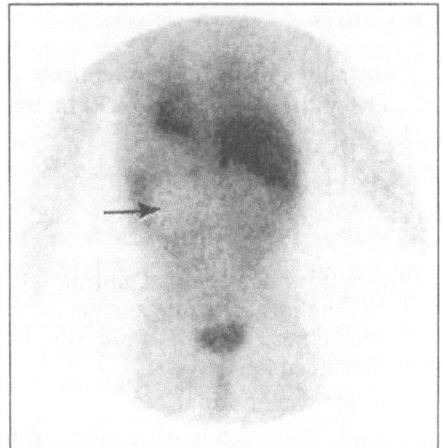

Fig. 5.8.vii. Posterior chest and abdomen

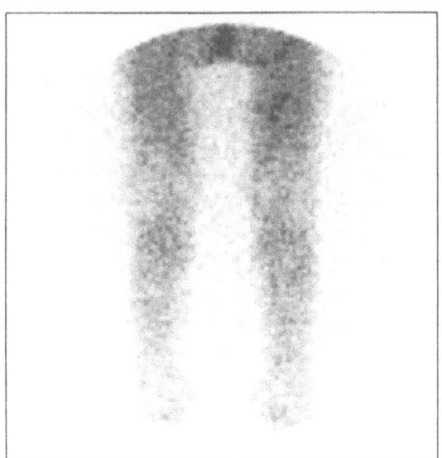

Fig. 5.8.viii. Posterior of legs

Isotope	123I
Activity given	185 MBq
Acquisition time per image	10 minutes
Collimator	low energy
Time of scan	24 hours

continued

Subsequent Course

In January 1988 after completing six courses of modified OPEC chemotherapy (Appendix F) he was reinvestigated.

Investigations

Abdominal ultrasound and abdominal and chest CT scans showed that the large, heterogeneous (solid, cystic and calcified) mass arising from the left adrenal had not changed in size.

Bone marrow studies were normal.

The ^{123}I-mIBG study (Figs. 5.8.ix–xi) continued to show a photon-deficient area at the site of the primary tumour. All other sites of disease which had previously shown increased uptake of mIBG, were now negative.

Comment

In view of the lack of change in size, and the lack of uptake of mIBG by the primary site, it was postulated that the primary site may be ganglioneuromatous tissue, despite malignant neuroblastoma cells being present in the bone marrow at diagnosis. The primary site was completely excised in February 1988, and histopathology revealed a smooth thin-walled cyst, filled with haemorrhagic debris, islands of intact adrenal parenchyma and sympathetic ganglia. No evidence of neuroblastoma was seen.

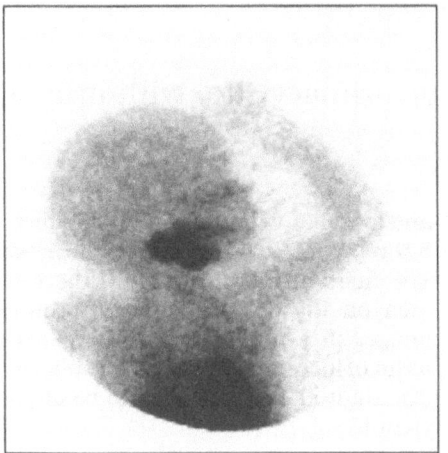

Fig. 5.8.ix. Right lateral skull

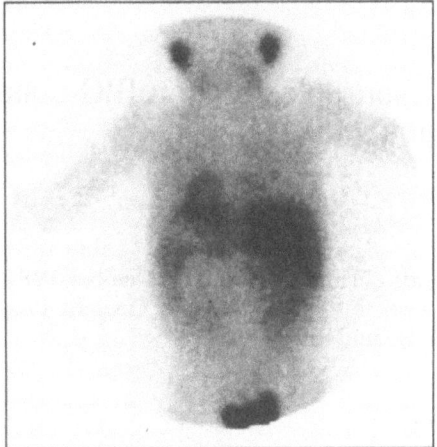

Fig. 5.8.x. Posterior chest and abdomen

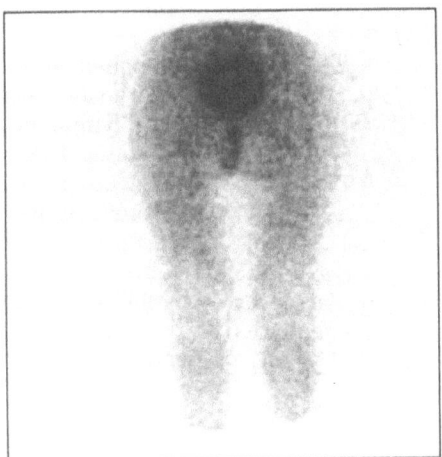

Fig. 5.8.xi. Posterior pelvis and legs

Isotope	123I
Activity given	185 MBq
Acquisition time per image	10 minutes
Collimator	low energy
Time of scan	24 hours

Stage IV Neuroblastoma: mIBG-negative primary site, with mIBG-positive focal bone metastases

History

This 20-month-old male presented in October 1987 with a six-week history of anorexia, weight loss, general malaise and irritability.

Investigations

A 24-hour urine collection showed raised levels of catecholamines.

Abdominal ultrasound and abdominal and chest CT scan showed a large partially calcified mass occupying the right upper abdomen, extending across the midline and displacing the right kidney into the right iliac fossa.

^{99m}Tc-MDP bone scans and bone marrow studies were normal.

The ^{123}I-mIBG study (Figs. 5.9.i–iv) showed increased uptake of mIBG in the soft tissue of the left side of the neck (Fig. 5.9.i, arrowed). There was also increased uptake in the nasopharyngeal area just to the right of the midline (Fig. 5.9.ii, arrow), and focal bony uptake in the right distal femur (Fig. 5.9.iv). There was no uptake in the bone marrow. The mass in the right side of the upper abdomen seen on the CT scan and ultrasound scans was imaged as a photon-deficient area, surrounded by a rim of increased mIBG uptake (Fig. 5.9.iii, arrow). The right kidney was seen to be displaced into the right iliac fossa.

Comment

This patient has stage IV neuroblastoma with the primary site arising from the right adrenal gland, and a lymph node metastasis and cortical bone metastasis. The mIBG-positive lymph node in the neck was excised and shown to contain neuro-blastoma. As in Case 8 the primary site does not take up mIBG, whereas the secondary sites have retained the ability to take it up. This raises the possibility that the histopathology of the primary site and the secondary sites may show different degrees of differentiation.

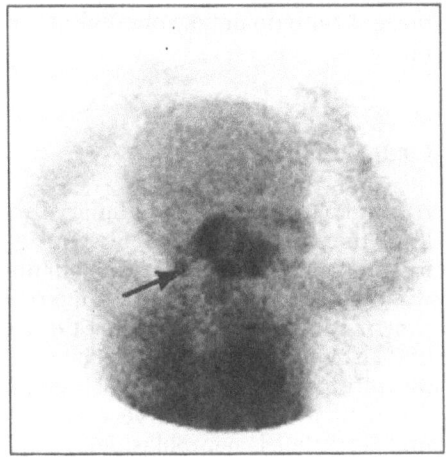

Fig.5.9.i. Right lateral skull

Fig. 5.9.ii. Posterior skull

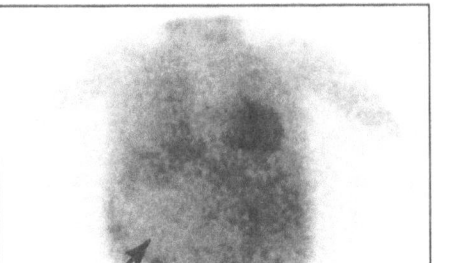

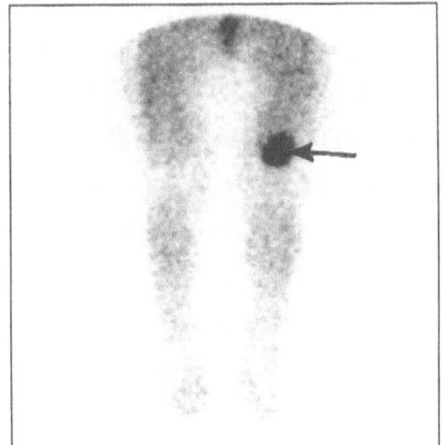

Fig. 5.9.iii. Anterior chest and abdomen

Fig. 5.9.iv. Posterior of legs

Isotope	123I
Activity given	185 MBq
Acquisition time per image	10 minutes
Collimator	low energy
Time of scan	24 hours

Subsequent Course

The child was treated with six courses of modified OPEC chemotherapy (Appendix F), and then re-investigated.

Investigations

A 24-hour urine collection showed lower levels of catecholamines.

Abdominal ultrasound and abdominal and chest CT scans showed a 75% reduction in the size of the primary tumour.

Bone marrow studies were normal.

The ^{123}I-mIBG examination (Figs 5.9.v–viii) was normal, with no uptake of mIBG at the primary site (arrows).

Comment

A subtotal excision of the primary tumour showed that the major component was ganglioneuroblastoma, with only a very small minor component containing undifferentiated tumour. It has been shown (Moyes et al. 1988) that the degree of mIBG uptake by neuroblastoma correlates with the quantity of undifferentiated neuroblastoma present. In this patient, there was a very small percentage of undifferentiated neuroblastoma, explaining why the primary site was mIBG-negative.

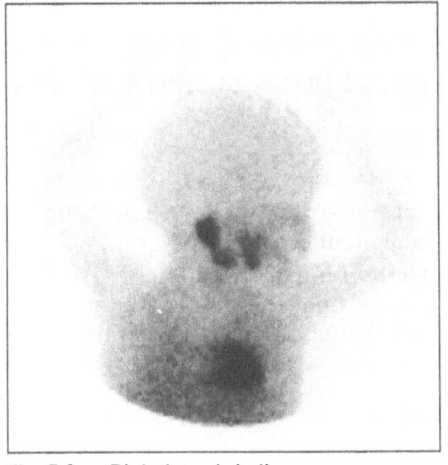

Fig. 5.9.v. Right lateral skull

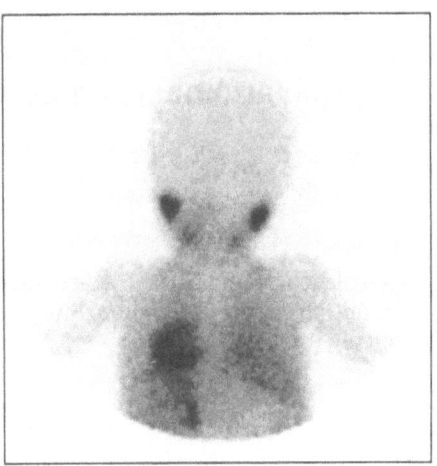

Fig. 5.9.vi. Posterior skull

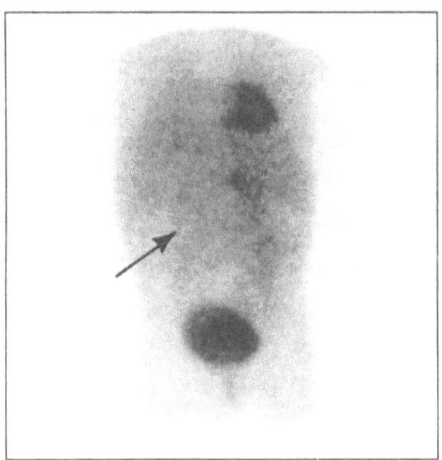

Fig. 5.9.vii. Anterior chest and abdomen

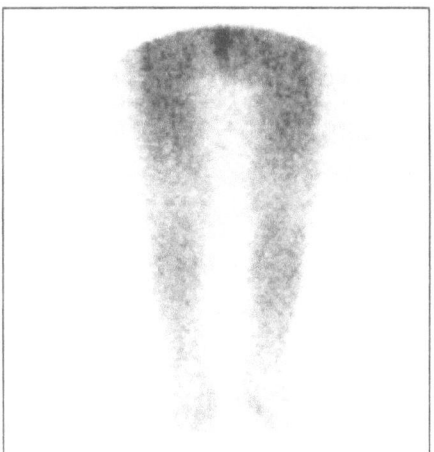

Fig. 5.9.viii. Posterior of legs

Isotope	123I
Activity given	185 MBq
Acquisition time per image	10 minutes
Collimator	low energy
Time of scan	24 hours

Stage IVs Neuroblastoma: left adrenal gland primary site with liver involvement

History

This 4-month female was found to have a distended abdomen on routine physical examination. She was otherwise extremely well.

Investigations

A 24-hour urine collection showed raised levels of catecholamines.

Abdominal and chest CT scans showed a massively enlarged liver with a large tumour arising from the left adrenal gland, and an enlarged lymph node in the left para-aortic region.

Bone marrow studies showed no infiltration by malignant cells.

The ^{123}I-mIBG study (Figs. 5.10.i–iii) showed increased uptake of mIBG in the abdomen. There were no other abnormal areas of mIBG uptake.

Comment

The increased uptake of mIBG into the massively enlarged liver can be clearly seen; however, the left adrenal tumour cannot be distinguished as a separate site of disease. This child has stage IVs neuroblastoma. The area of increased activity seen in the right wrist (Fig. 5.10.i) is the site of intravenous injection of the radiopharmaceutical.

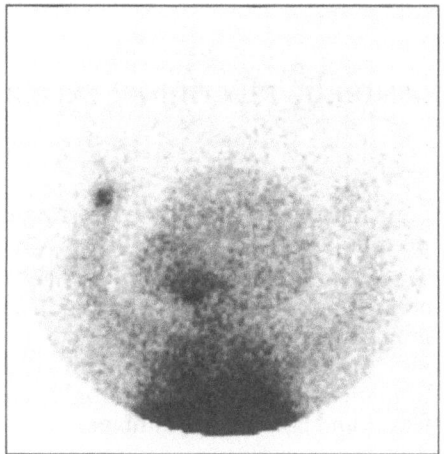

Fig.5.10.i. Left lateral skull

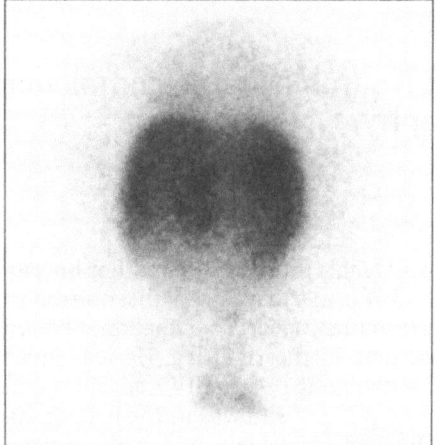

Fig. 5.10.ii. Posterior chest and abdomen

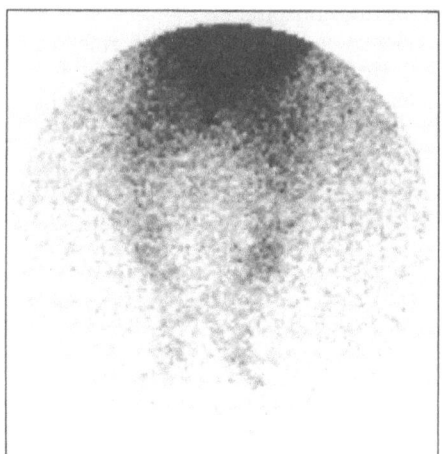

Fig. 5.10.iii. Posterior of legs

Isotope	^{123}I
Activity given	75 MBq
Acquisition time per image	10 minutes
Collimator	low energy
Time of scan	24 hours

Stage IV Neuroblastoma: complete remission by all criteria, except mIBG scintigraphy

History

This 6½-year-old male presented to another hospital in September 1986, aged 5 years, with a one month history of intermittent fever, constipation, abdominal pain and pain in the right leg. He was investigated and a diagnosis of stage IV neuroblastoma was made. The primary site was in the left adrenal gland and he had focal bone and bone marrow metastases. He was treated with chemotherapy, followed by complete excision of the primary site. He was then reinvestigated at the referring hospital and it was felt that there was no evidence of disease (an mIBG study was not performed). He was therefore referred to The Royal Marsden Hospital for re-evaluation prior to total body irradiation and autologous bone marrow rescue. He was then reinvestigated in April 1987.

Investigations

A 24-hour urine collection showed marginally raised levels of catecholamines.

Bone marrow studies at the referring hospital were normal.

The ^{123}I-mIBG study (Figs. 5.11.i–iv) showed increased uptake of mIBG in the bone marrow of the long bones, pelvis and vertebral column. There was also focal bony uptake in both orbits, proximal humeri, iliac wings and proximal femora, left distal femur and both proximal tibiae.

Comment

At the referring hospital mIBG scintigraphy had not been performed, and therefore this patient was thought to be in complete clinical remission. However, the ^{123}I-mIBG scan shows intense uptake of mIBG in the cortical bone and bone marrow consistent with neuroblastoma involvement at these sites.

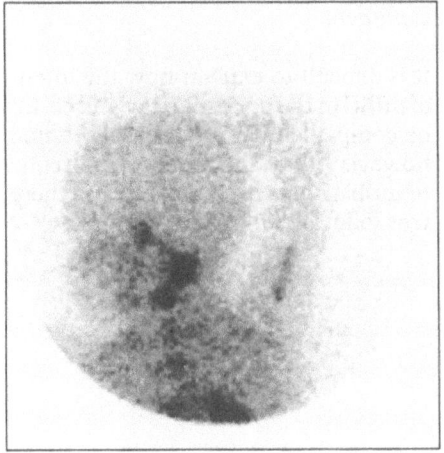

Fig.5.11.i. Left lateral skull

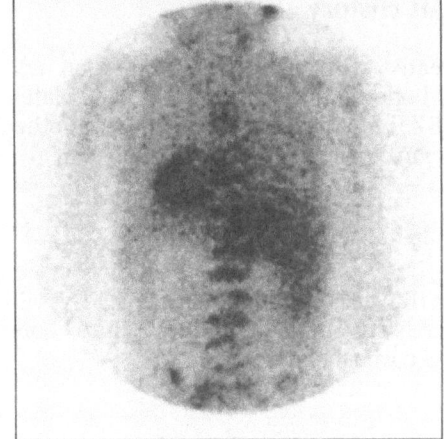

Fig. 5.11.ii. Posterior chest and abdomen

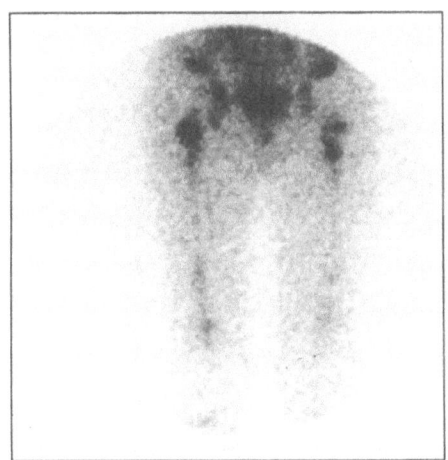

Fig. 5.11.iii. Posterior of upper legs

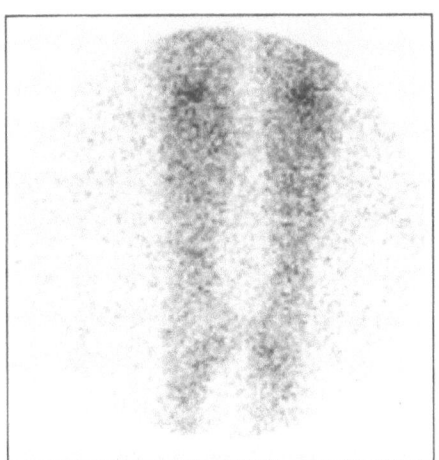

Fig. 5.11.iv. Posterior of lower legs

Isotope	^{123}I
Activity given	185 MBq
Acquisition time per image	10 minutes
Collimator	low energy
Time of scan	24 hours

continued

Subsequent History

He was treated with total body irradiation and autologous bone marrow rescue. Six weeks later, in May 1987, he was reinvestigated with another ^{123}I-mIBG scan.

Investigations

The ^{123}I-mIBG scintigrams (Figs. 5.11.v–viii) showed persistent uptake of mIBG into bone marrow and cortical bone.

Comment

It is difficult to explain how the intensity of uptake of mIBG in the bone marrow and cortical bone could be compatible with a disease-free state. It was felt, however, that the uptake did represent residual neuroblastoma at these sites, and therefore the child was followed up closely.

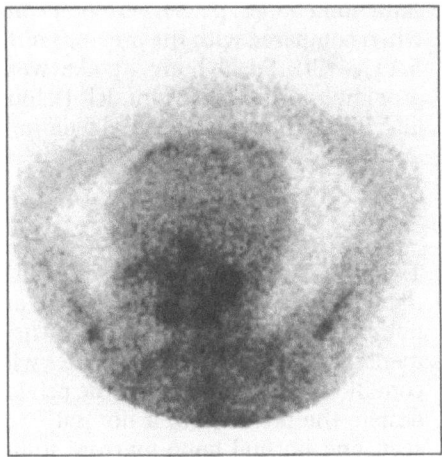

Fig. 5.11.v. Left lateral skull

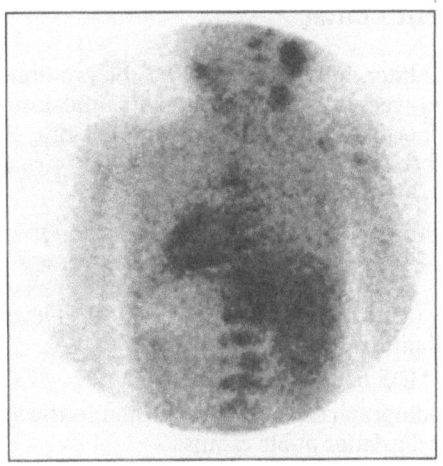

Fig. 5.11.vi. Posterior chest and abdomen

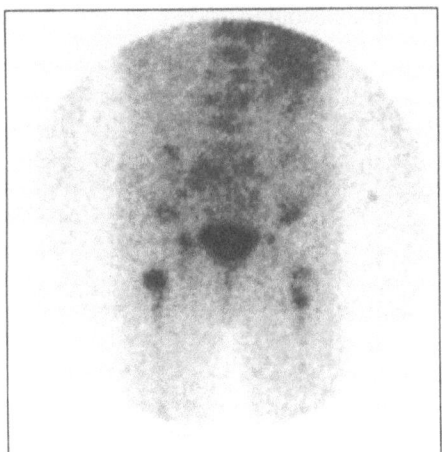

Fig. 5.11.vii. Posterior abdomen and pelvis

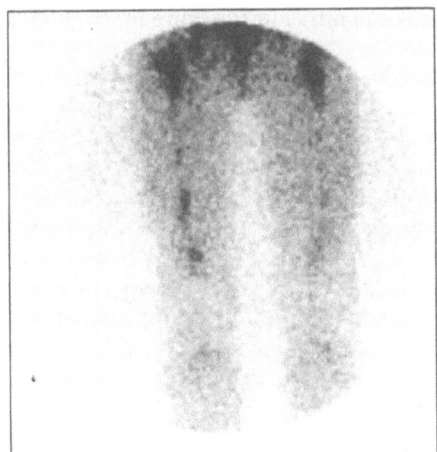

Fig. 5.11.viii. Posterior of upper legs

Isotope	^{123}I
Activity given	185 MBq
Acquisition time per image	10 minutes
Collimator	low energy
Time of scan	24 hours

continued

Subsequent Course

Six months later, in November 1987, he presented with a one-week history of irritability and intermittent bone pain, particularly of the left hip. He was therefore reinvestigated.

Investigations

A 24-hour urine collection showed increased levels of catecholamines.

The ^{99m}Tc-MDP bone scan was normal.

A pelvic radiograph showed a lytic lesion in the left ischium and inferior pubic ramus.

Bone marrow studies were normal.

The ^{123}I-mIBG study (Figs 5.11.ix–xii) showed more intense uptake of mIBG in the bone marrow of the skull, long bones, pelvis, vertebral column and ribs, when compared with the previous mIBG study (Figs 5.11.v–viii). Focal bony uptake was seen in the proximal humeri, sternum, left ischium, left sacroiliac joint, and both proximal femora.

Comment

The mIBG study indicates widespread bone marrow uptake of the radiopharmaceutical, and focal bony uptake at the site of clinical pain. The mIBG assessment of the disease state correlates with the clinical condition of the patient and the pelvic radiographs, despite the presence of a normal ^{99m}Tc-MDP bone scan and normal bone marrow studies. The bone marrow studies were repeated two weeks later, and this time showed widespread involvement with neuroblastoma.

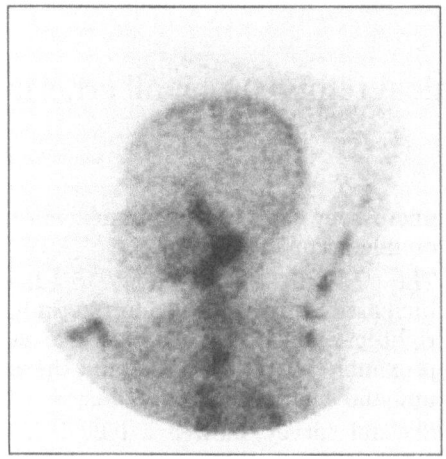

Fig. 5.11.ix. Left lateral skull

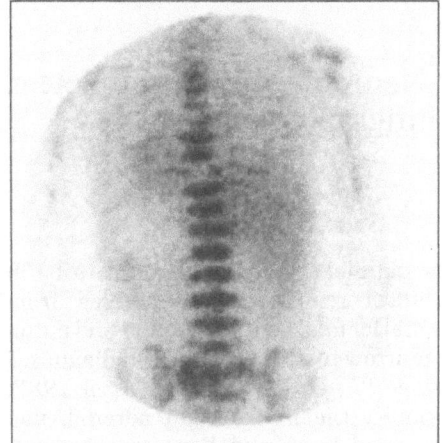

Fig. 5.11.x. Posterior chest and abdomen

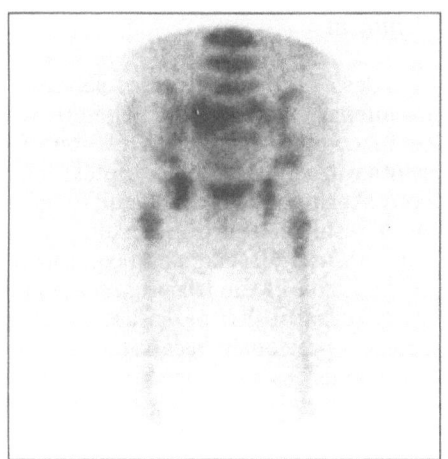

Fig. 5.11.xi. Posterior pelvis and upper legs

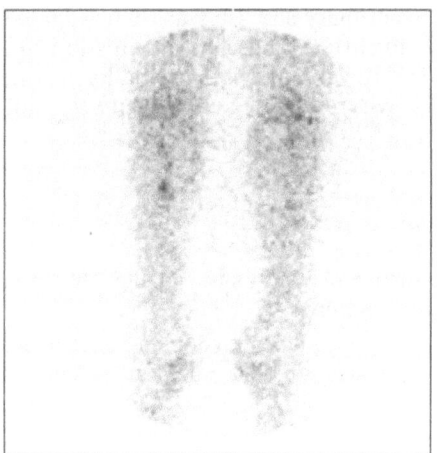

Fig. 5.11.xii. Posterior of lower legs

Isotope	123I
Activity given	185 MBq
Acquisition time per image	10 minutes
Collimator	low energy
Time of scan	24 hours

Stage IV Neuroblastoma: complete clinical remission by all criteria, except mIBG scintigraphy

History

This $3\frac{1}{2}$ year old male who was thought to be in complete clinical remission was referred from another hospital for total body irradiation and autologous bone marrow rescue. He had been diagnosed as having stage IV neuroblastoma in April 1987, with the primary site in the right adrenal, and lymph node, focal bone and bone marrow secondaries. He was treated with OPEC chemotherapy (Appendix A), and had macroscopically complete excision of his primary site. He was reinvestigated, assessed as being in complete clinical remission, and referred to The Royal Marsden Hospital for further treatment. He was restaged to verify complete clinical remission.

Investigations

A 24-hour urine collection showed slightly raised levels of catecholamines.

Bone marrow studies were inconclusive with one clump of suspicious cells demonstrated on microscopy of aspirates, but no abnormality shown on microscopy of trephines.

The ^{123}I-mIBG study (Figs. 5.12.i–iv) showed increased uptake of mIBG in the skull, both orbits, right proximal humerus, thoracic vertebrae, left proximal and distal femur, and the proximal end and mid-shaft of the right tibia.

Skeletal survey showed a lytic lesion in the left proximal femur.

Comment

Like Case 11, this child was referred to our hospital for intensification therapy when he was thought to be in complete clinical remission. The ^{123}I-mIBG scintigram shows intense uptake of mIBG in the bony skeleton, which is difficult to regard as normal. As a result of the mIBG examination, a skeletal survey was undertaken and confirmed the presence of the lesion in the left proximal femur. The mIBG study revealed sites of disease which had not been detected previously because mIBG studies had not been done.

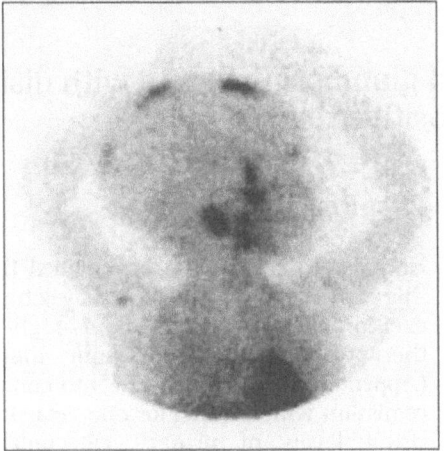

Fig.5.12.i. Right lateral skull

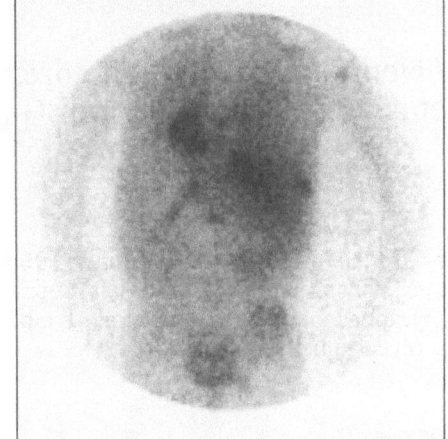

Fig. 5.12.ii. Posterior chest and abdomen

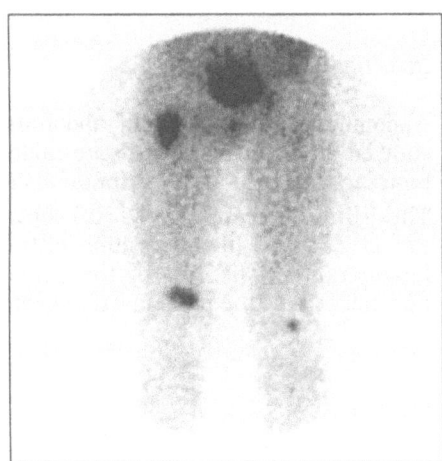

Fig. 5.12.iii. Posterior of upper legs

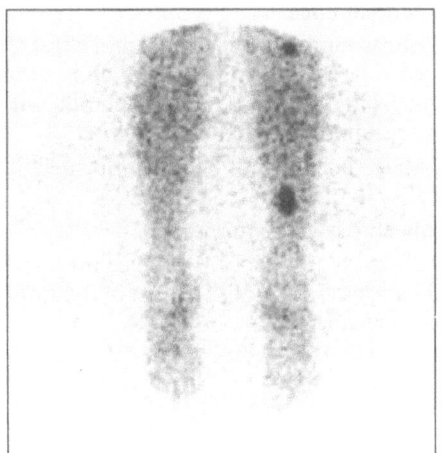

Fig. 5.12.iv. Posterior of lower legs

Isotope	^{123}I
Activity given	185 MBq
Acquisition time per image	10 minutes
Collimator	low energy
Time of scan	24 hours

Stage IV Neuroblastoma: right adrenal gland primary site with distal lymph node metastases; followed by mIBG-positive relapse

History

An $8\frac{1}{2}$-year-old male presented in December 1984 with a large abdominal mass and left supra-clavicular lymphadenopathy. Excisional lymph node biopsy revealed neuroblastoma.

Investigations

A 24-hour urine collection showed markedly raised levels of catecholamines.

Abdominal ultrasound and abdominal and chest CT scans showed a large right-sided upper abdominal mass arising from the right adrenal gland, with associated para-aortic lymphadenopathy.

The ^{99m}Tc-MDP bone scan showed no definite abnormality.

Bone marrow studies were normal.

The ^{131}I-mIBG study (Fig. 5.13.i) showed increased uptake in the para-aortic area. The rest of the mIBG examination was normal.

Comment

The ^{131}I-mIBG scan shows intense uptake in the very large abdominal tumour. The normal body landmarks are difficult to identify as the ^{131}I isotope has been used.

First Relapse

He received six courses of modified OPEC chemo-therapy (Appendix F), followed by complete surgical excision of the adrenal tumour, high-dose chemo-therapy and autologous bone marrow rescue (Appendix B). He then went into complete clinical remission which lasted for one year. In June 1986 rising levels of urinary catecholamines were detected.

Investigations

Abdominal ultrasound and abdominal CT scans showed an abnormal soft-tissue nodal mass lying between the aorta and inferior vena cava.

The ^{123}I-mIBG scan (Fig. 5.13.ii) showed increased uptake of mIBG in the position of the para-aortic lymph nodes. The rest of the examination was normal, as was the bone marrow examination.

Comment

Full re-staging showed the para-aortic nodes to be the only site of relapse, and the ^{123}I-mIBG scan shows intense uptake at this site, with preservation of normal body landmarks (cf. Fig. 5.13.i)

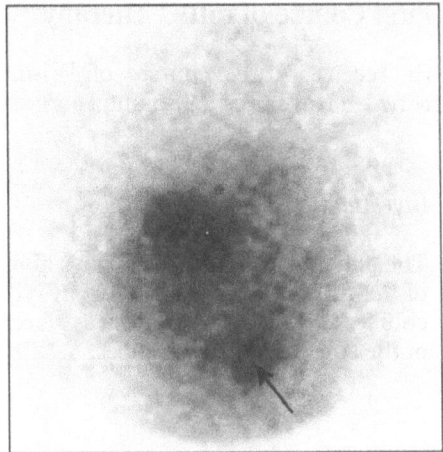

Fig.5.13.i. Anterior abdomen

Isotope	^{131}I
Activity given	18 MBq
Acquisition time per image	5 minutes
Collimator	high energy
Time of scan	48 hours

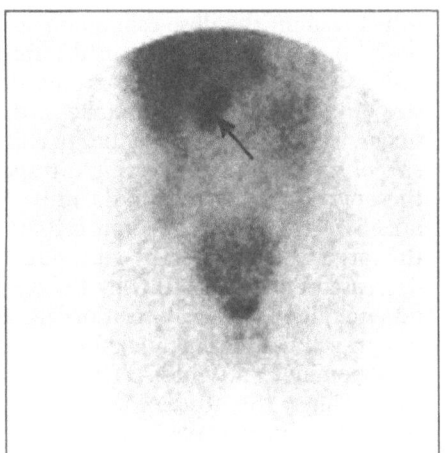

Fig. 5.13.ii. Anterior abdomen and pelvis

Isotope	^{123}I
Activity given	185 MBq
Acquisition time per image	5 minutes
Collimator	low energy
Time of scan	24 hours

continued

Second Relapse

The para-aortic lymph nodes were completely excised. In October 1986 the patient represented with recurrent para-aortic lymphadenopathy.

Investigations

A 24-hour urine collection for catecholamines was normal.

Abdominal and chest CT scans showed recurrent nodal disease around the inferior vena cava, and metastases in the liver.

An abdominal ultrasound examination showed para-aortic lymphadenopathy around and extending into the inferior vena cava. The liver appeared to be normal.

Bone marrow investigations were normal.

The ^{131}I-mIBG study (Fig. 5.13.iii) showed increased uptake of mIBG in the para-aortic area, and also in a patchy distribution throughout the liver.

Comment

The ^{131}I isotope was used on this occasion for the purpose of dosimetry estimations, since it was planned that the patient would go on to receive targetted radiotherapy with mIBG.

First Course of mIBG Therapy

He received three courses of ^{131}I-mIBG therapy between November 1986 and February 1987.

Investigations

The patient was scanned six days after each course of ^{131}I-mIBG therapy (Figs. 5.13.iv–vi). For the first course 2.7 GBq of ^{131}I-mIBG was given and for each of the subsequent two courses, 3.7 GBq was given.

Comment

The liver and para-aortic nodal relapse took up mIBG well on the dose-estimation scintigram (Fig. 5.13.iii). Scans after each of the three courses of mIBG therapy showed a progressive decrease in the size of the area of mIBG uptake in the para-aortic nodes. This could be due either to a decrease in the size of the tumour, indicating a response to mIBG therapy, or an alteration in the mIBG uptake mechanism of the neuroblastoma cells (as a result of the targetted radiotherapy with mIBG) resulting in decreased uptake of mIBG by the tumour. The left adrenal gland is clearly seen on Fig. 5.13.iv when a high-activity therapeutic dose has been given.

Abdominal and chest CT scans performed four weeks after the third course of mIBG therapy showed complete resolution of the para-aortic lymphadenopathy, with only one liver metastasis remaining visible.

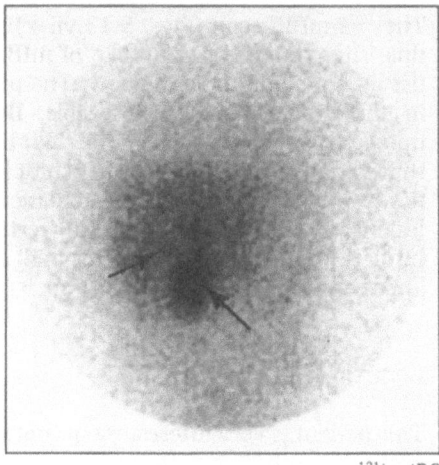

Fig. 5.13.iii. Anterior abdomen. At 72 hours after administration of diagnostic activity (October 1986).

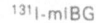

Fig. 5.13.iv. Anterior abdomen. At 6 days after administration of therapy activity (November 1986).

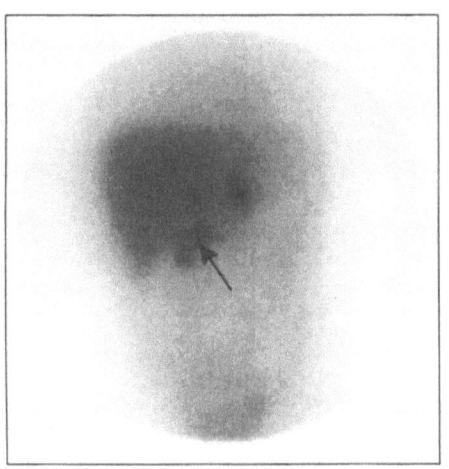

Fig. 5.13.v. Anterior abdomen. At 6 days after administration of therapy activity (December 1986).

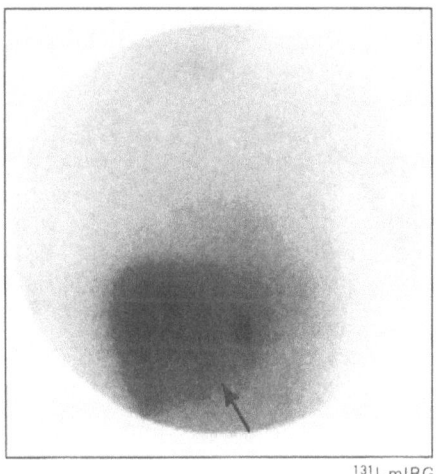

Fig. 5.13.vi. Anterior chest and abdomen. At 6 days after administration of therapy activity (February 1987).

continued

119

Third Relapse

As a result of the mIBG therapy, the patient suffered severe thrombocytopenia requiring platelet transfusions. Otherwise he remained extremely well until June 1987 when he was reinvestigated because a 24-hour urine collection showed rising levels of catecholamines.

Investigations

Abdominal and chest CT scans showed multiple small rounded opacities in both lung fields consistent with metastatic disease. In the abdomen there was a soft-tissue mass in the region of the head of the pancreas, and para-aortic lymphadenopathy.

The ^{99m}Tc-MDP bone scan was normal.

Bone marrow studies showed infiltration with neuroblastoma.

The ^{123}I-mIBG scan (Figs. 5.13.vii–x) showed multiple sites of increased uptake of mIBG in the soft tissue, bone and bone marrow. The patchy uptake in the lungs was clearly visible. Bone marrow uptake was demonstrated in the right humerus, and thoracic and lumbar vertebrae. Multiple sites of soft-tissue uptake were seen in the abdomen. Focal bony lesions were seen in the skull vertex, proximal humeri, right proximal femur and around both knees.

Comment

This patient is very interesting in that the recurrent areas of neuroblastoma have retained the ability to take up mIBG, despite having previously been treated with the radiopharmaceutical. The bone marrow uptake, however, is less obvious than that seen in other patients (cf. Figs. 5.3.i–iv) who have not received mIBG therapy.

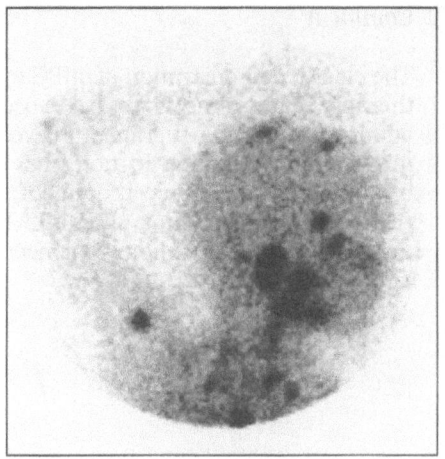

Fig. 5.13.vii. Right lateral skull

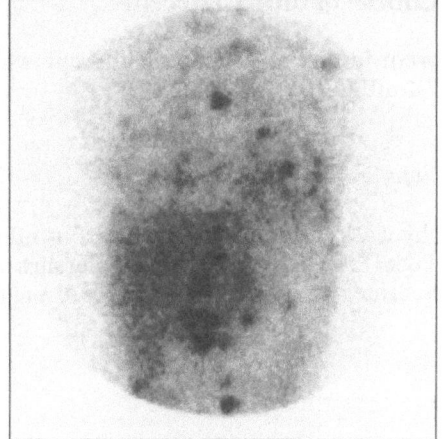

Fig. 5.13.viii. Anterior chest and abdomen

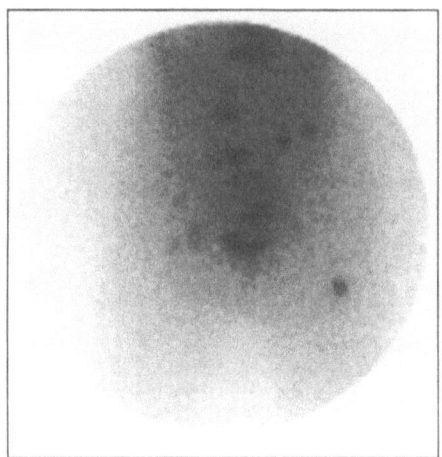

Fig. 5.13.ix. Posterior abdomen and pelvis

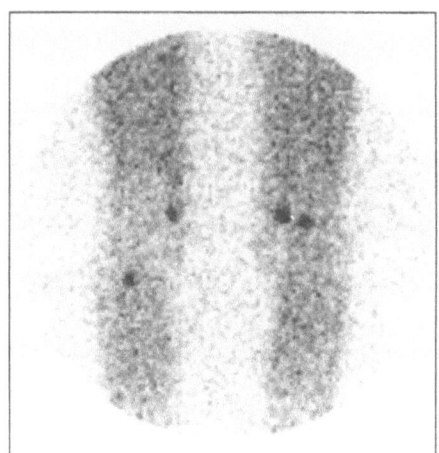

Fig. 5.13.x. Posterior of legs

Isotope	^{123}I
Activity given	185 MBq
Acquisition time per image	10 minutes
Collimator	low energy
Time of scan	24 hours

continued

Second Course of mIBG Therapy

He underwent further targetted radiotherapy with 5.4 GBq ^{131}I-mIBG.

Investigations

Scintigraphy was performed six days after ^{131}I-mIBG therapy (Figs. 5.13.xi–xiv). The multiple sites of disease illustrated in Figs. 5.13.vii–x were again shown.

Comment

The clearer demonstration of mIBG uptake on these therapy scintigrams is to be expected after the administration of a therapeutic level of activity of mIBG. It is interesting to note that bone marrow uptake is still not very prominent. This may be related to the fact that after mIBG therapy, the ability of recurrent tumour to concentrate mIBG is altered.

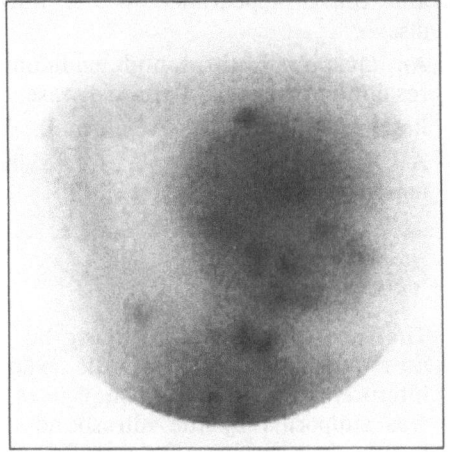

Fig. 5.13.xi. Right lateral skull

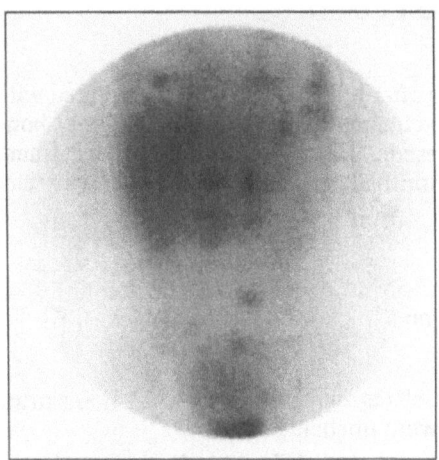

Fig. 5.13.xii. Anterior abdomen

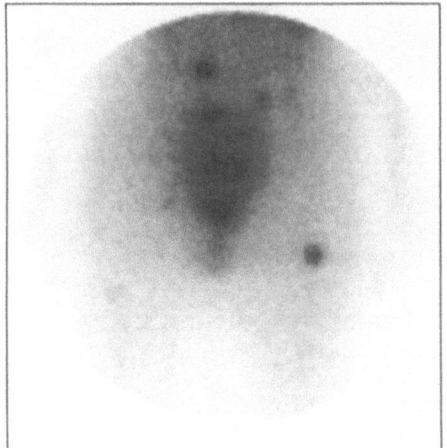

Fig. 5.13.xiii. Posterior pelvis

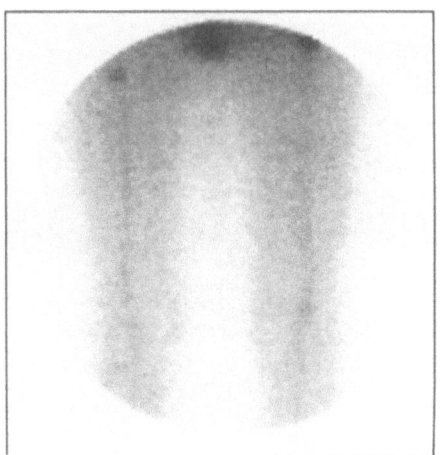

Fig. 5.13.xiv. Posterior of upper legs

Isotope	^{131}I
Activity given	5.4 GBq
Acquisition time per image	10 minutes
Collimator	high energy
Time of scan	6 days

continued

Subsequent Course

Two weeks after mIBG therapy he was treated with high-dose chemotherapy and autologous bone marrow rescue. He responded to this treatment and two months later (September 1987) was reinvestigated.

Investigation

The levels of catecholamines in a 24-hour urine collection were unchanged.

Abdominal and chest CT scans showed resolution of all the previously visible pulmonary metastases and the disappearance of the intra-abdominal disease.

An abdominal ultrasound examination showed resolution for the para-aortic disease.

Bone marrow studies were normal.

A ^{123}I-mIBG study (Figs. 5.13.xv–xviii) showed no abnormal areas of uptake of mIBG.

Comment

The sites which had previously taken up mIBG, no longer do so, and the mIBG examination was interpreted as indicating complete remission. This was supported by the ultrasound and CT scan results. Increased uptake of mIBG is seen in the indwelling right atrial catheter in Figs. 5.13.xv–xvi.

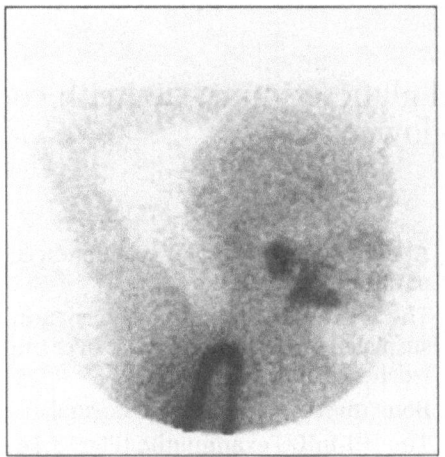
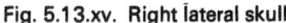

Fig. 5.13.xv. Right lateral skull

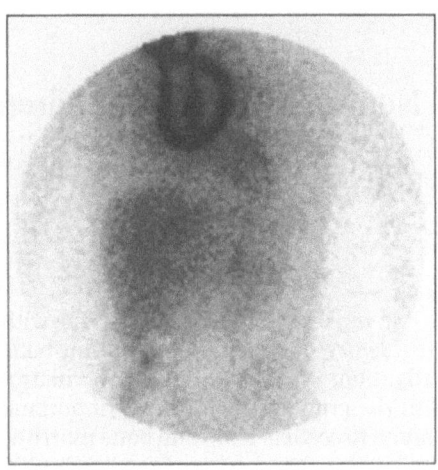

Fig. 5.13.xvi. Anterior chest and abdomen

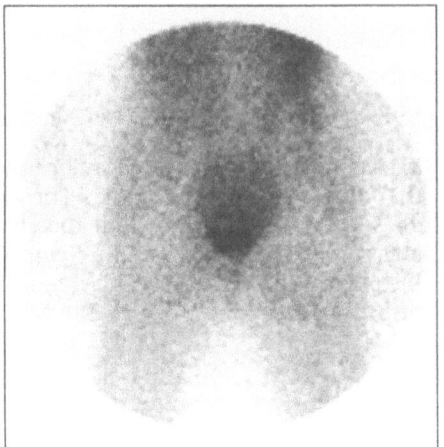

Fig. 5.13.xvii. Posterior pelvis

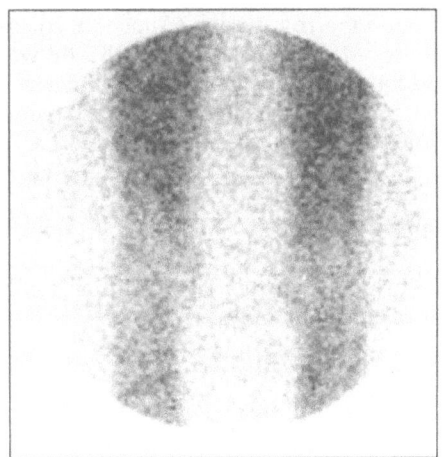

Fig. 5.13.xviii. Posterior of upper legs

Isotope	^{123}I
Activity given	185 MBq
Acquisition time per image	10 minutes
Collimator	low energy
Time of scan	24 hours

Stage IV Neuroblastoma: right adrenal gland primary site with cortical bone and bone marrow metastases; followed by mIBG-negative relapse

History

This 9½-year-old male presented in July 1984 with a one month history of abdominal pain and bone pain. Investigations revealed stage IV neuroblastoma with the primary site in the right adrenal gland and spread to cortical bone and bone marrow. He was treated with seven courses of modified OPEC chemotherapy (Appendix F), complete surgical excision of the primary site, high-dose melphalan and autologous bone marrow rescue (Appendix B). At the completion of treatment in June 1985 he was restaged and found to have no evidence of disease. In September 1986 he was referred back with recurrent chest infections, and was reinvestigated.

Investigations

A 24-hour urine collection showed marginally raised levels of catecholamines.

Abdominal and chest CT scans showed a right-sided para-aortic soft-tissue mass.

The ^{99m}Tc-MDP bone scan was equivocal, with a suspicion of increased activity over the right greater trochanter.

Bone marrow studies were normal.

The ^{123}I-mIBG examinaton (Figs. 5.14.i–iv) showed no abnormal areas of uptake of mIBG.

Comment

Excisional biopsy of the para-aortic mass showed that this was neuroblastoma. The site of relapse does not take up mIBG, and therefore represents a false-negative mIBG study. Some patients with histologically proven neuroblastoma do not take up mIBG, the aetiology of which has not been clarified.

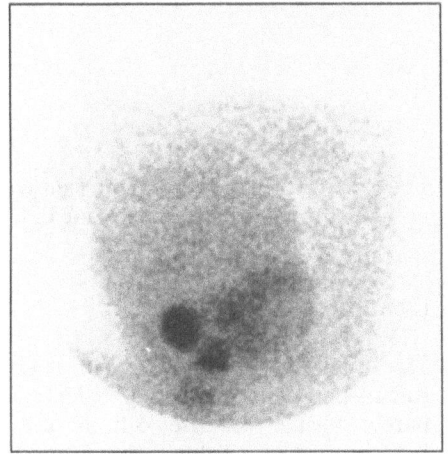

Fig.5.14.i. Right lateral skull

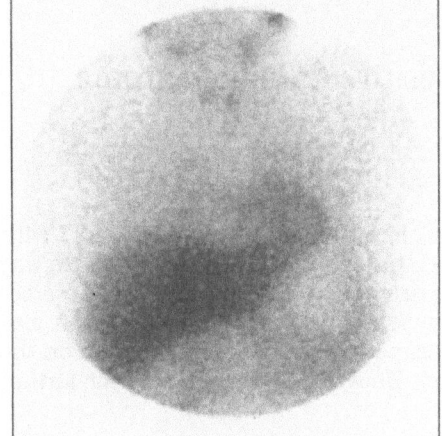

Fig. 5.14.ii. Anterior chest

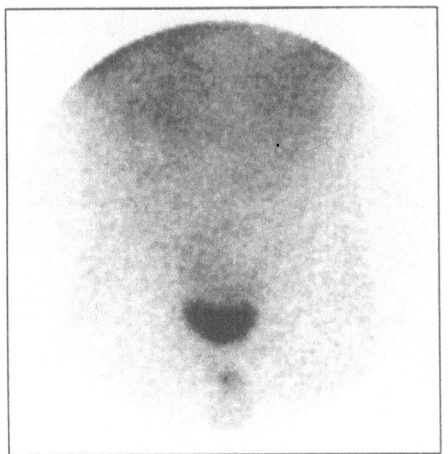
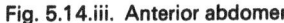

Fig. 5.14.iii. Anterior abdomen

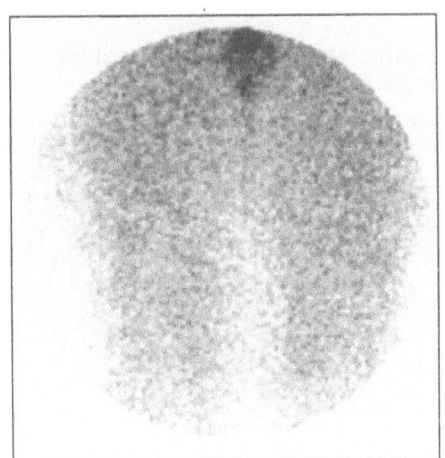

Fig. 5.14.iv. Anterior of upper legs

Isotope	^{123}I
Activity given	185 MBq
Acquisition time per image	10 minutes
Collimator	low energy
Time of scan	24 hours

mIBG-positive Ganglioneuroma

History

This 6-year-old male presented in April 1987 with a three-week history of a persistent cough. He was otherwise extremely well. On a routine chest radiograph (Figs. 5.15.i–ii) a rounded mass lesion was seen in the superior, posterior mediastinum on the left (arrows). He was therefore referred for further assessment.

Investigations

A 24-hour urine collection showed raised levels of catecholamines.

Abdominal and chest CT scans showed a left-sided, round soft-tissue mass in the posterior mediastinum.

Bone marrow studies were normal.

The ^{123}I-mIBG (Fig. 5.15.iv) showed increased uptake of mIBG in the upper zone of the left lung.

Comment

The uptake into the chest lesion is clearly seen on the 24-hour scintigram (Fig. 5.15.iv, arrow), but is barely visible on the 4-hour scintigram (Fig. 5.15.iii, arrow). Taking the clinical history and the results of all the investigations into consideration, a diagnosis of ganglioneuroma or ganglioneuroblastoma is the most likely.

Subsequent course

Complete surgical excision of the mass revealed the histopathology to be ganglioneuroma.

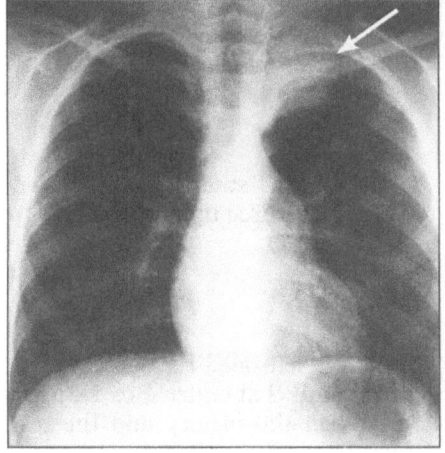

Fig.5.15.i. Anterior chest

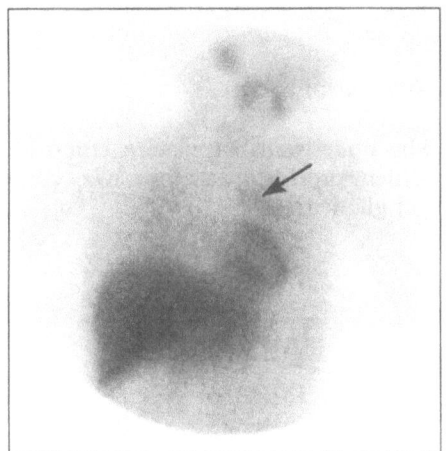

Fig. 5.15.ii. Lateral chest

4 hours
Fig. 5.15.iii. Anterior chest

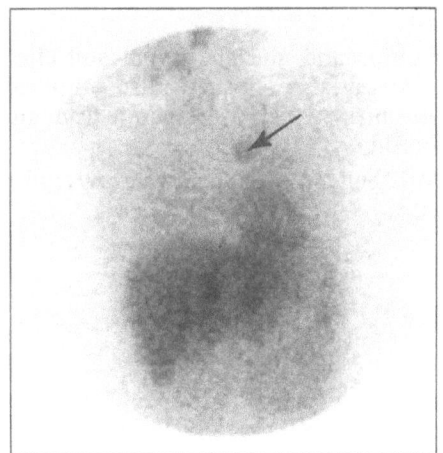

24 hours
Fig. 5.15.iv. Anterior chest

Isotope	123I
Activity given	185 MBq
Acquisition time per image	10 minutes
Collimator	low energy

mIBG-negative Ganglioneuroma

History

This $4\frac{1}{2}$-year-old female presented in July 1987 with a history of intermittent abdominal pain of several years' duration. She was otherwise completely well. Physical examination revealed a left-sided abdominal mass.

Investigations

The levels of urinary catecholamines were marginally raised.

Abdominal ultrasound and abdominal and chest CT scan showed a large left-sided retroperitoneal, heterogeneous mass, which was separate from and medial to the kidney.

The ^{99m}Tc-MDP bone scan and bone marrow studies were normal.

The ^{123}I-mIBG study (Figs. 5.16.i–iv) showed no areas of increased uptake of mIBG.

Comment

The large left-sided retroperitoneal mass does not take up mIBG at either 4 or 24 hours, unlike Case 15. When the history and the results of all the investigations (including the raised catecholamines) are taken into account, the most likely diagnosis is a ganglioneuroma.

Subsequent course

She underwent complete excision of the tumour, which on histopathology was shown to be a ganglioneuroma.

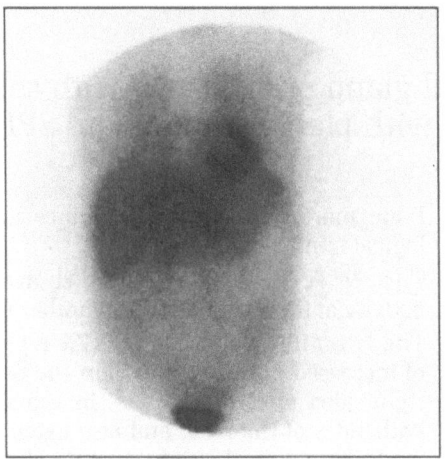

4 hours

Fig. 5.16.i. Anterior chest and abdomen

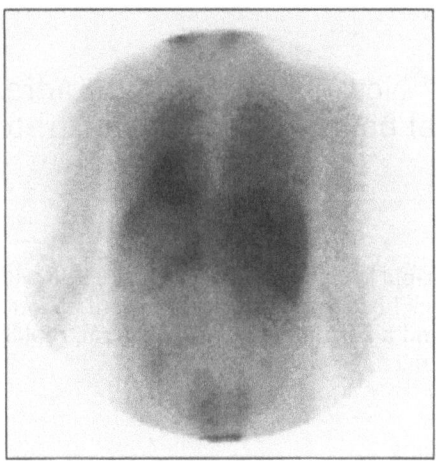

4 hours

Fig. 5.16.ii. Posterior chest and abdomen

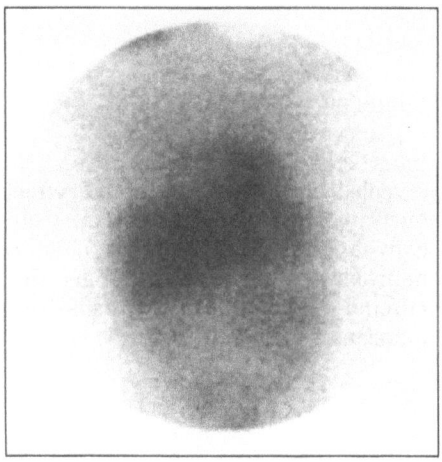

24 hours

Fig. 5.16.iii. Anterior chest and abdomen

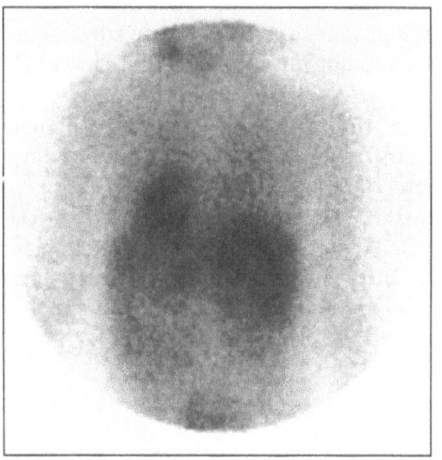

24 hours

Fig. 5.16.iv. Posterior chest and abdomen

Isotope	^{123}I
Activity given	185 MBq
Acquisition time per image	10 minutes
Collimator	low energy

Stage IV Neuroblastoma: right adrenal gland primary site with soft-tissue and focal bone metastases, illustrated with planar images and SPECT

History

This 9-year-old female presented in April 1988 with a three-week history of left upper quadrant abdominal pain, and a 24-hour history of bilateral, rapidly enlarging, neck nodes.

Investigations

A 24-hour urinary collection showed markedly raised levels of catecholamines.

A chest radiograph showed a mediastinal mass which was extending up into the right side of the neck.

Ultrasound of the neck and abdomen showed masses on both sides of the neck, and a large heterogeneous right-sided abdominal mass.

CT scans of the neck, chest and abdomen showed bilateral cervical lymphadenopathy, with extension on the right into the mediastinum. A very large right-sided abdominal mass which extended across the midline was also seen.

Bone marrow aspirates, trephines and immunological markers were normal.

The ^{99m}Tc-MDP bone scan showed increased activity at the site of the third lumbar vertebra (L3). The ^{123}I-mIBG study (Figs. 5.17.i–iv) showed areas of increased uptake of mIBG in the predominantly right-sided abdominal mass, in the soft tissue on both sides of the neck and also extending into the mediastinum on the right. Increased activity is also seen in the upper lumbar vertebrae (L1, L2 and L3). There was no uptake of mIBG into the bone marrow.

Comment

In a single investigation the ^{123}I-mIBG study revealed all the sites of disease which were demonstrated by a combination of techniques using conventional methods. This child has stage IV neuroblastoma with the primary site in the right adrenal gland and distant soft-tissue and bone metastases.

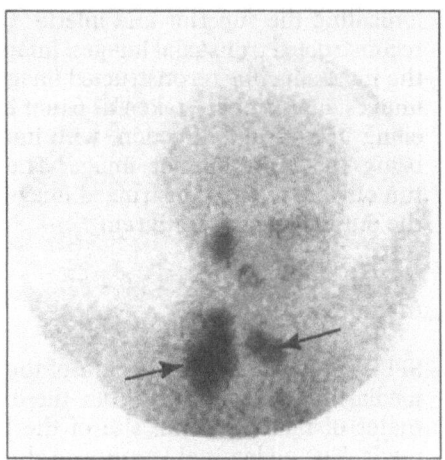

Fig.5.17.i. Right lateral skull

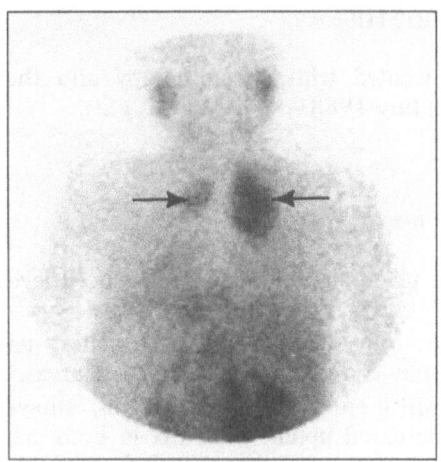

Fig. 5.17.ii. Posterior chest and abdomen

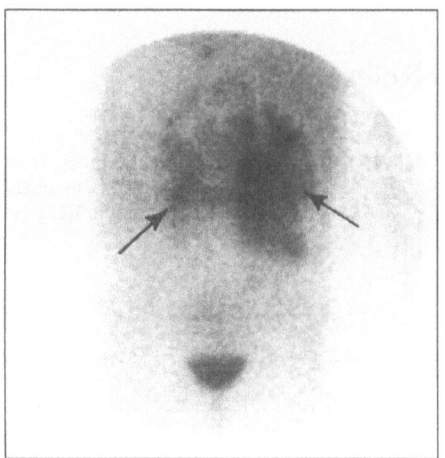

Fig. 5.17.iii. Posterior abdomen and pelvis

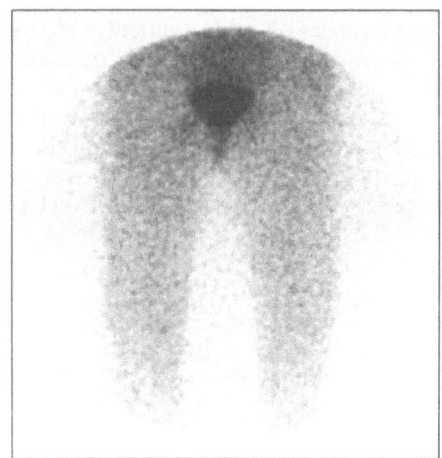

Fig. 5.17.iv. Posterior pelvis and upper legs

Isotope	^{123}I
Activity given	185 MBq
Acquisition time per image	10 minutes
Collimator	low energy
Time of study	24 hours

continued

Subsequent History

She was treated with chemotherapy and then restaged in July 1988.

Investigations

A 24-hour urine collection showed reduced levels of catecholamines.

Ultrasound and CT scans of neck, chest and abdomen showed residual disease in these areas.

The ^{123}I-mIBG study (Figs. 5.17.v–viii) showed residual increased uptake of mIBG in both sides of the neck and mediastinum, and the abdomen (arrows). In order to delineate the lesions in the mediastinum and abdomen more accurately SPECT was also performed on this patient. Figures 5.17.x(a–l) show the reconstructed transaxial images which demonstrate the upper and lower boundaries of the mediastinal lesion, as well as giving an impression of its three-dimensional shape. The planar scintigram (Fig. 5.17.ix) shows the lesion in the mediastinum, with the horizontal lines indicating the superior and inferior borders of the reconstructed transaxial images. Image 5.17.x(a) is the most superior reconstructed image, and all the images after that are taken at 6 mm intervals travelling in a caudal direction, with image 5.17.x(1) being the most inferior image. The area of the tumour on each reconstructed image is shown by the outline on the scintigram.

Comment

SPECT studies show the extent of the lesion in the mediastinum very well. From these images, estimates of the functional size of the lesion can be made. The abdominal lesion was also equally well delineated by SPECT.

Reference

Moyes JSE, Babich JW, Carter R et al. (1988). Quantitative measurement of uptake of mIBG in children with neuroblastoma (Nb). Nucl Med Commun 9:175–176.

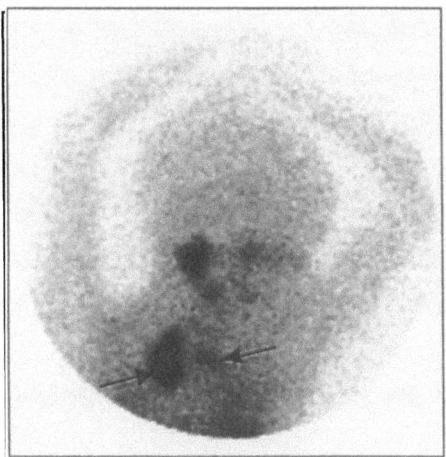

Fig. 5.17.v. Right lateral skull

Fig. 5.17.vi. Posterior chest

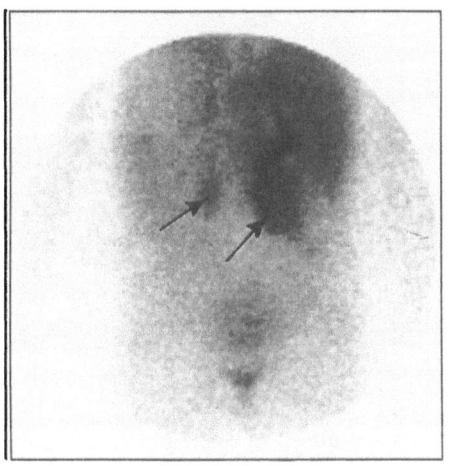

Fig. 5.17.vii. Posterior abdomen and pelvis

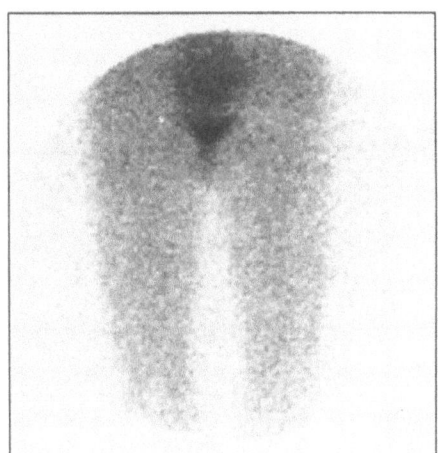

Fig. 5.17.viii. Posterior pelvis and upper legs

Isotope	^{123}I
Activity given	185 MBq
Acquisition time per image	10 minutes
Collimator	low energy
Time of scan	24 hours

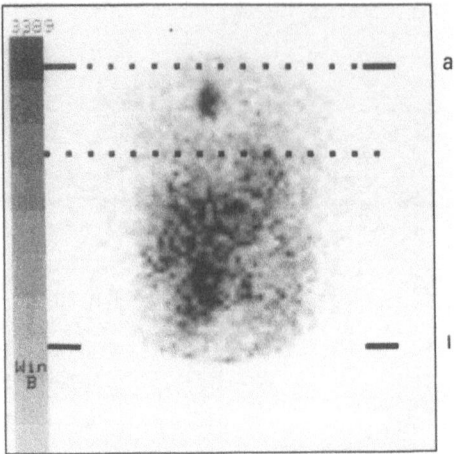

Fig. 5.17.ix. Anterior chest and abdomen

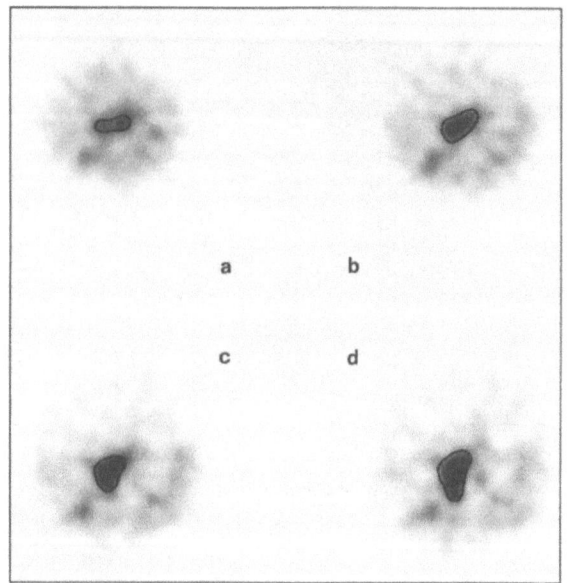

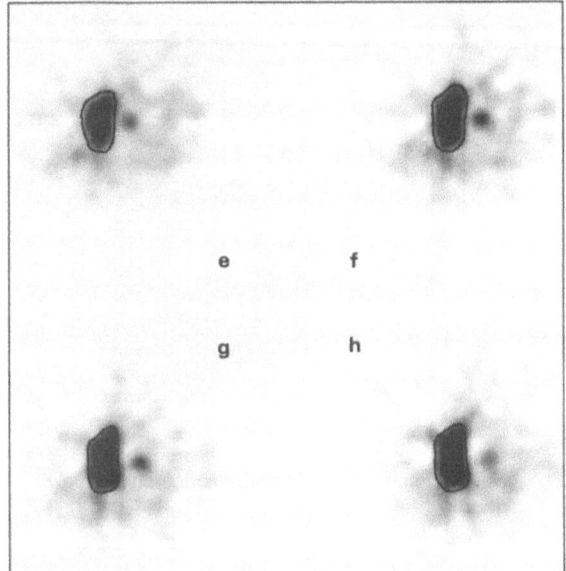

Fig. 5.17.x(a,b,c,d). Transaxial images

Fig. 5.17.x(e,f,g,h). Transaxial images

Fig. 5.17.ix and x. SPECT study
The planar image (Fig. 5.17.ix) shows the lesion in the mediastinum, with the horizontal lines indicating the superior and inferior borders of the reconstructed transaxial images. Images 5.17.x(a–l) represent transaxial scintigrams taken at 6 mm intervals travelling in a cephalo–caudal direction. The borders of the tumour are outlined as shown.

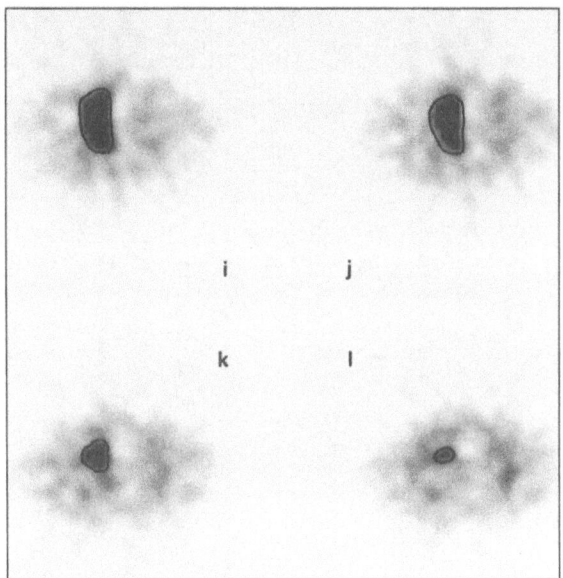

Fig. 5.17. x (i,j,k,l). Transaxial images

SPECT	
Isotope	^{123}I
Activity given	185 MBq
Acquisition time per image	20 seconds
Collimator	low energy
Time of study	24 hours

6 Radiation Dosimetry of Radioiodine-labelled mIBG

Sue L. Fielding and Maggie A. Flower

When radiation interacts with matter, the energy of the radiation is transferred to the atoms of the material through which it passes. The ionisation and excitation caused by the interaction of radiation give rise to biological effects which can produce damage to the cell (chromosomal aberrations, mutation), damage to tissue (transformation of cells to a malignant state), or a whole-body damaging effect.

The absorbed radiation dose in matter is the energy deposited per unit mass by ionising radiations, and the techniques for calculating the absorbed dose have become widely accepted. It is important to calculate the absorbed dose to the whole body and to various body organs in order to evaluate the radiation risk to a patient from the diagnostic use of radioiodine-labelled mIBG. The small risk of biological effects must be balanced against the potential benefit to the patient from the information obtained. In radiotherapy, the radiation dose to the whole body, or to tissues other than the tumour, may be the limiting factor. Hence, when ^{131}I-labelled mIBG is administered therapeutically, it is essential that the radiation dose to the whole body, and to other individual organs be determined.

Review of Radionuclide Dosimetry

Estimates of the radiation dose which will be delivered by any radioactive isotope introduced into the body can be made using the techniques recommended by the Committee on Medical Internal Radiation Dose (MIRD) of the American Society of Nuclear Medicine. The MIRD system (reviewed by Schlesinger 1978) uses the units of rad and curie (Ci), but for use in this chapter these have been converted to SI units of gray (Gy) and megabecquerels (MBq). Other SI units used are mass in grams (g), time in hours (h) and effective dose equivalent in millisievert (mSv) (Paić 1988).

When a radionuclide is administered internally it will distribute throughout the whole body and accumulate in various organs. When calculating absorbed doses from internal radiation, it is necessary to separate the various organs and radioactive distributions involved. For example, with radioiodine-labelled mIBG, the absorbed dose to the liver will be the sum of the dose due to activity in the liver, plus the dose due to activity in the rest of the body which irradiates the liver. The organ containing the radioactivity is referred to as the source

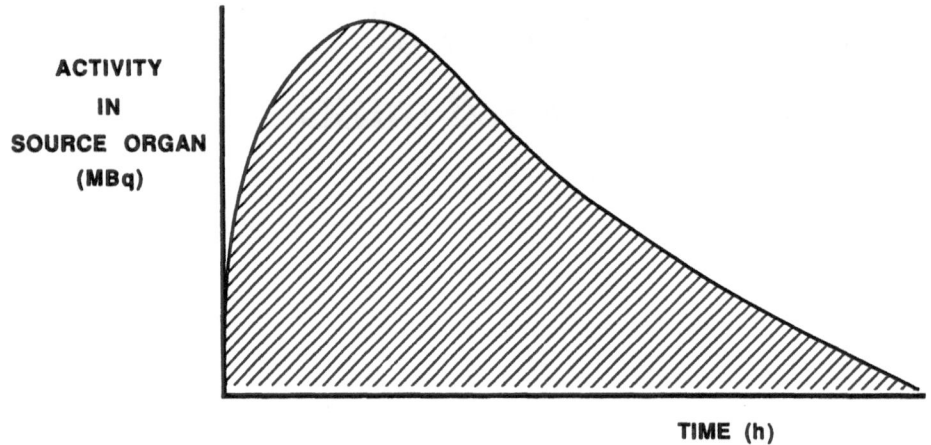

Fig. 6.1. Activity in a source organ as a function of time. The shaded area represents the cumulated activity.

organ (s) and the organ being irradiated is called the target organ (t).

The basic equation for the absorbed dose to a target organ (t) from activity in a source organ (s) can be expressed as:

$$D_t = \frac{\tilde{A}}{m_t} \times \sum_i (\Delta_i \times \varphi_i) \qquad (1)$$

where D_t = absorbed dose to target organ (Gy),

$\tilde{A}$ = cumulated activity in source organ (MBq·h),

Δ_i = dose constant for the ith type radiation, i.e. the rate the energy is emitted from the source organ per unit activity (g·Gy/MBq·h),

φ_i = fraction of ith type radiation emitted from the source organ which is absorbed by the target organ,

m_t = mass of the target organ (g),

$\sum_i$ = the sum of $\Delta_i \times \varphi_i$, for all values of i.

Cumulated activity, $\tilde{A}$

The cumulated activity, $\tilde{A}$, gives the total number of radioactive disintegrations which occur in the source organ. $\tilde{A}$ is determined by the administered activity, the uptake of activity into the source organ, excretion from the organ and the physical decay of the radiolabel.

Figure 6.1 shows a typical graph of activity in a source organ against time. The cumulated activity, $\tilde{A}$, is represented by the shaded area under the curve. Often the uptake into an organ is so rapid that the initial part of the curve can be ignored. Hence, an appropriate mathematical description of

the pharmacokinetic behaviour of the radiopharmaceutical can be given by one or more exponential functions.

For a single exponential function, the cumulated activity is given by:

$$\tilde{A} = 1.44 \times A_0 \times T_e \qquad \text{in MBq·h} \qquad (2)$$

where A_0 = initial uptake in the source organ (MBq),

T_e = effective half-life (h) of the radiopharmaceutical in that organ.

The effective half-life (T_e) of a radiopharmaceutical is a combination of the physical half-life of the radiolabel, T_p, and the biological half-life of the pharmaceutical, T_b. The physical half-life of the radiolabel is the time for an amount of radioactivity to decay naturally to one half of its original value. The biological half-life of the pharmaceutical is the time for the amount of the pharmaceutical to be reduced to one half of its original value by excretion from the organ of interest. The relationship between these different half-lives is given by:

$$\frac{1}{T_e} = \frac{1}{T_p} + \frac{1}{T_b} \qquad (3)$$

Very often, the clearance of activity from an organ can be shown to have two or three exponential components. In order to separate out the exponential components, two methods can be used. Either curve stripping techniques, which enable the true effective half-lives of each component to be assessed, or a simpler technique which enables the assessment of apparent effective half-lives. The latter technique is based on the assumption that the activity–time curve, as plotted on log–linear graph paper, can be approximated to two or three straight lines. Figure 6.2 shows a whole-body time–activity

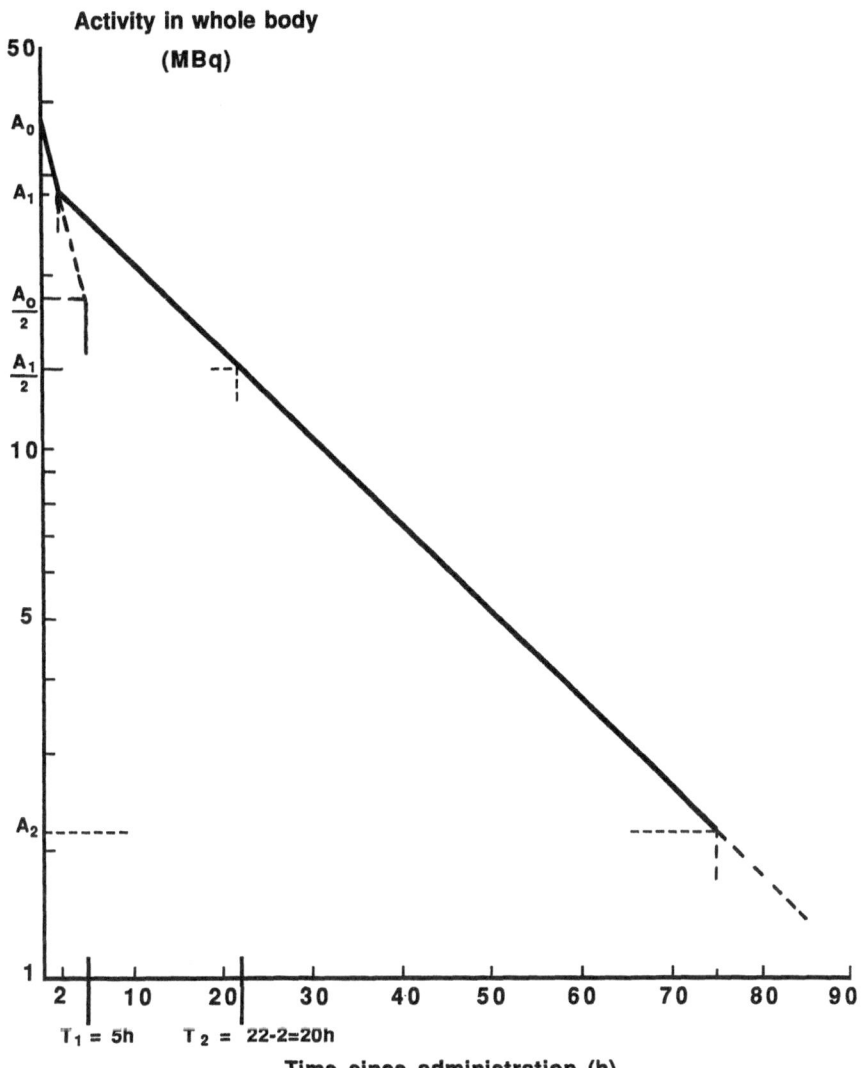

Fig. 6.2. Whole-body activity as a function of time from a diagnostic study performed with ^{131}I-mIBG (plotted on log–linear graph paper). The apparent effective half-life of the early fast component (T_1) is marked (*5h*). The effective half-life of the second slower component (T_2) is the time taken for the activity A_1 to decrease to $A_1/2$ as shown on the graph. The last measured activity is A_2 at 75 hours

curve, which has been approximated to two straight lines.

In this example, the cumulated activity is given by:

$$\bar{A} = 1.44 \times \{[(A_0 - A_1) \times T_1] + (A_1 \times T_2)\} \quad (4)$$
$$\text{in MBq} \cdot \text{h}$$

where A_0 = the initial activity (MBq)

A_1 = the activity (MBq) at that point on the graph where the two straight lines intersect,

T_1 = the apparent effective half-life (h) of the early fast phase component,

T_2 = the effective half-life (h) of the later slower component.

Equilibrium dose constant, Δ_i

The radiolabel may emit non-penetrating radiation (beta rays) as well as penetrating radiation (gamma rays, X-rays). Each type of radiation has a value Δ_i associated with it, which is the amount of energy released in that form per disintegration. Values of Δ_i are tabulated for most radionuclides used in nuclear medicine (MIRD 1975a).

Absorbed fraction, φ_i

The absorbed fraction is the ratio of the energy absorbed in the target organ to the total energy

141

Table 6.1. The physical properties of ^{131}I and [123]I.

	Physical half-life	Non-penetrating				Penetrating			
	(h)	Rad'n	E* (keV)	Δ (g·Gy/MBq·h)	%	Rad'n	E (keV)	Δ (g·Gy/MBq·h)	%
[123]I	13.0	—	—	—	—	$\gamma1$	159	0.077	83.6
						$\gamma9$	529	0.003	1.1
[131]I	193.4	$\beta1$	69.0	0.008	2.0	$\gamma4$	284	0.010	5.8
		$\beta3$	96.4	0.004	6.6	$\gamma9$	364	0.172	82.0
		$\beta5$	191.6	0.099	89.8	$\gamma12$	637	0.023	6.5
						$\gamma14$	723	0.007	1.7

E*, mean β energy: E, γ energy.
From MIRD (1975a).

emitted by the radioactivity in the source organ.

$$\varphi_i = \frac{\text{energy of type } i \text{ absorbed in target organ}}{\text{energy of type } i \text{ emitted from source organ}}$$
(5)

For non-penetrating radiation, the absorbed fraction is unity for cases where the source organ is also the target organ, and zero for all other cases. For penetrating radiation, only partial absorption occurs in the source organ and in the surrounding tissues and organs. MIRD Pamphlet 5 (MIRD 1969) gives data from computer calculations performed to assess the absorbed fractions for a variety of radionuclides and organs of Reference Man, weight 70 kg.

Mean dose per unit cumulated activity, S

All of the physiological data needed for the estimation of dose are contained in the cumulated activity $\bar{A}$. The remaining portion of equation (1) involves physical and anatomical data only. The MIRD technique introduces the quantity S, the absorbed dose per unit cumulated activity (Gy/MBq·h)

$$S_{(s \to t)} = \sum_i (\Delta_i \times \Phi_i)$$
(6)

where Δ_i = equilibrium dose constant for the ith type radiation,

Φ_i = the specific absorbed fraction for the ith type radiation ($= \varphi_i/m_t$).

Thus, the total absorbed dose to a target organ (t) from a single source organ (s) is:

$$D_t = \bar{A} \times S_{(s \to t)}$$
(7)

For a number of source organs, the total dose is simply equal to the sum of the individual doses from each source organ.

S-values have been tabulated for various source–target configurations and various radionuclides commonly used in nuclear medicine (MIRD 1975b). The MIRD values assume the activity is uniformly distributed in the source organ, and the phantom used for estimating the absorbed fractions is essentially that used in MIRD Pamphlet 5 (MIRD 1969), which was designed to represent Reference Man. The S-values depend on the radiation characteristics of the radionuclide, the absorption of the various radiation types in different tissues, and the assumed physical dimensions of the organs considered.

The Physical Properties of ^{123}I and [131]I

The two isotopes mainly used as radiolabels for mIBG are ^{123}I and [131]I. Each has different physical properties so that, although both forms of radioiodine-labelled mIBG may be used for scanning purposes, only ^{131}I-labelled mIBG is used for targetted radiotherapy.

Table 6.1 illustrates the physical properties of these two radioisotopes of iodine and gives the energies of the most abundant radiations. The low energy (159 keV) of the ^{123}I photons makes this radioisotope particularly suitable for use with a gamma camera. Typical values for detection efficiency and spatial resolution are 91% (for a half-inch crystal) and 5 mm at 5 cm depth, respectively. A total of 83.6% of the emissions are of 159 keV gamma rays and the radionuclide can be considered to be mono-energetic. Emissions from the radioisotope can be efficiently collimated with a low-energy collimator (e.g. one designed to have < 5% penetration at 180 keV). The radionuclide emits the minimum of non-penetrating emissions (as its decay is via electron capture) and has a short physical half-life of 13 hours. These physical properties result in a low radiation dose for ^{123}I-mIBG with the effective dose equivalent being 7 mSv per 400 MBq administered isotope (ARSAC 1988). Thus, ^{123}I is the radionuclide of choice for diagnostic use.

[131]I emits both beta and gamma rays. The main beta energy of 192 keV, and the longer physical half-life of 8.06 days (193.4 hours) make the radioisotope suitable for targetted radiotherapy. The penetrating gamma ray emissions can also be used for imaging purposes, but ^{131}I is not an ideal radionuclide for imaging. Typical values for detection efficiency and spatial resolution are 30% (for a half-inch crystal) and 10 mm at 5 cm depth, respectively. The main energy of emitted gamma rays is 364 keV but, even with a high-energy collimator (e.g. one designed to have < 5% penetration at 380 keV), the photons emitted at 637 and 723 keV penetrate through the collimator and shielding. The higher equilibrium dose constants, and the presence of non-penetrating radiations result in a higher radiation dose to individual organs for ^{131}I compared with [123]I. The effective dose equivalent for ^{131}I-mIBG is 4 mSv per 20 MBq administered isotope (ARSAC 1988).

Calculation of Absorbed Dose in Children

Dose Received in Diagnostic Studies

The methods for calculating the absorbed dose to individual organs from administered mIBG are the same for both radioisotopes, but the appropriate S-values must be used in the calculations.

Table 6.2. Organ weights for paediatric and adult phantoms

Organ	Weight (g)			
	Newborn	1 yr	5 yr	Adult
Liver	110	300	608	1809
Kidneys	19	68	116	284
Thyroid	1	2	5	20
Lungs	40	130	260	1000
Whole body	3990	10400	20000	70000

Reproduced in part with permission from NCRP (1983).

S-values

Since most cases of neuroblastoma occur in the younger age range, the majority of patients being injected with radio-iodine-labelled mIBG are children. Thus the S-values for both ^{123}I and ^{131}I need to be adapted for the size and weights of the organs of young children. The National Council on Radiation Protection and Measurements Report No. 73 (NCRP 1983) includes a section devoted to the estimation of absorbed radiation dose in paediatrics. The report presents an appendix with extensive tabulation of S-values derived from different paediatric phantoms. Several authors (Kereiakes et al. 1972; Poston 1976) provide information on body weights and organ weights and some typical values are shown in Table 6.2.

The S-values are higher in children than adults, and larger absorbed doses will be obtained in infants and children per MBq administered since the weights of body organs in children are smaller than those assumed for Reference Man. Table 6.3 lists some S-values to be used for newborn, 1-year-old, 5-year-old and adult patients injected with either [123]I- or ^{131}I-mIBG. The table shows S-values for configurations where both the source and target organs are either the whole body (WB), or the liver (L).

Table 6.3. Typical S-values for ^{123}I and [131]I (Gy/MBq·h)

	[123]I		[131]I	
	WB→WB	L→L	WB→WB	L→L
Newborn	1.01×10^{-5}	2.31×10^{-4}	3.76×10^{-5}	1.11×10^{-3}
1 year	4.46×10^{-6}	9.59×10^{-5}	1.55×10^{-5}	4.27×10^{-4}
5 year	2.52×10^{-6}	5.32×10^{-3}	8.43×10^{-6}	2.22×10^{-4}
Adult	8.38×10^{-7}	2.14×10^{-5}	2.68×10^{-6}	8.11×10^{-5}

From MIRD (1975b) and NCRP (1983).

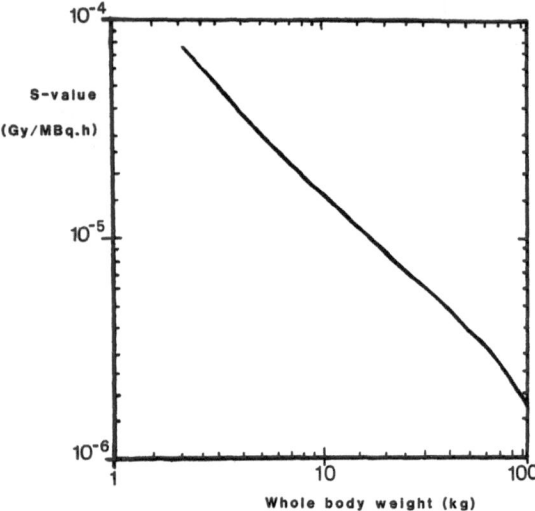

Fig. 6.3. Whole-body weight as a function of $S_{(WB \to WB)}$, plotted on log–log graph paper

To aid in the extrapolation needed when applying the dosimetry calculations to specific cases, graphs of S-values against organ weight are very useful. An example of the value of $S_{(WB \to WB)}$ against body weight is shown in Fig. 6.3.

Assessment of cumulated activity ($\tilde{A}$)

Several authors have described quantitative methods for the in-vivo measurement of radio-activity within an organ (Fleming 1979; Myers et al. 1981; Clarke et al. 1982). By placing regions of interest over the images of each source organ on conjugate views taken with a gamma camera (as shown in Fig. 6.4), estimates of the radioactivity accumulated in an organ can be made. This is obtained by comparing the counts within these regions of interest with the counts from a known amount of the radionuclide in a phantom of similar dimensions to those of the patient. Correction should be made for attenuation if the patient thickness and overall phantom thickness are not the same.

As shown in equation (3), the effective half-life of mIBG in an organ is determined by the biological elimination of the mIBG and the physical half-life of the radio-iodine used as the label. Sequential gamma-camera images can be made and the quantitative methods mentioned above can be used to assess activity in an organ at various times. The time required for the radioactivity in the organ to diminish by 50% is the effective half-life (T_e) and this can be determined from a graph of activity versus time (plotted on log–linear graph paper).

When considering the whole body as the source organ, the initial activity in the whole body is simply the activity injected. The activity remaining in the whole body at subsequent times can be obtained using a whole-body counter (e.g. a ceiling-mounted detector). If a reading is made immediately after injection, all future readings can be compared with that reading to give the activity in the whole body.

Figure 6.2 shows the whole-body clearance graph for a 5-year-old patient given 37 MBq ^{131}I-mIBG as part of a diagnostic study. The values were obtained at regular intervals using a ceiling-mounted detector. The effective half-lives of each component of the clearance curve can be obtained from the graph. From Fig. 6.2, 8.9 MBq ($A_0 - A_1 = 37 - 28.1$ MBq) of the mIBG is cleared by 2 hours with an apparent effective half-life of 5 hours. A further 25.9 MBq ($A_1 - A_2 = 28.1 - 2.2$ MBq) of the mIBG is cleared by 75 hours, with an effective half-life of 20 hours.

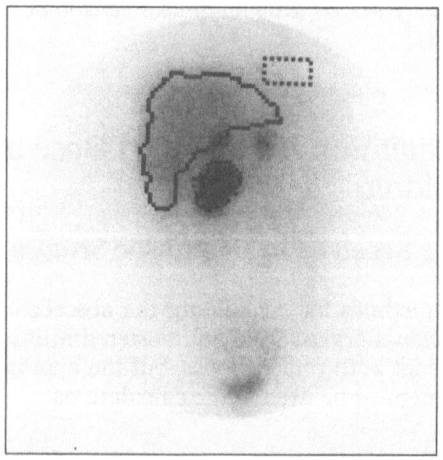

Fig. 6.4. mIBG scintigram showing regions of interest placed over the tumour, liver and a representative background area

Worked example

Using the data from Fig. 6.2, the whole-body to whole-body dose from an initial injection of 37 MBq of ^{131}I-mIBG can be calculated. From Table 6.3, the value of $S_{(WB \to WB)}$ for a 5-year-old child for ^{131}I is 8.43×10^{-6} Gy/MBq·h. Using equation (4) and substituting $A_0 = 37$ MBq, $A_1 = 28.1$ MBq, $T_1 = 5$ h and $T_2 = 20$ h, this gives:

$$\tilde{A} = 1.44 \times \{[(37-28.1) \times 5] + (28.1 \times 20)\}$$
$$= 1.44 \times (44.5 + 562)$$
$$= 873.36 \text{ MBq·h}$$

From equation (7),

$$D_{(WB \to WB)} = \tilde{A} \times S_{(WB \to WB)}$$
$$= 873.36 \times (8.43 \times 10^{-6}) \text{ Gy}$$
$$= 7.36 \times 10^{-3} \text{ Gy}$$
$$= 7.36 \text{ mGy}$$

The total whole-body to whole-body dose from 37 MBq of ^{131}I-mIBG is 7.36 mGy (0.20 mGy/MBq) in this example. This calculation assumes that the whole-body clearance continues with a half-life of 20 hours. Very often, a third slower phase is evident from around 70–150 hours after injection, and shows a third half-life (T_3) of approximately 60–120 hours (S. L. Fielding, 1987, unpublished data). To estimate the maximum dose possible from the data in Fig. 6.2, physical decay only can be assumed from 75 hours onwards. Adding a third component to equation (4), and using $A_2 = 2.2$ MBq and $T_3 =$ the physical half-life of [131]I $= 8.06$ days (193.4 h), the equation becomes:

$$\tilde{A} = 1.44 \times \{[37-28.1) \times 5] + [(28.1-2.2) \\ \times 20] + (2.2 \times 193.4)\}$$
$$= 1.44 \times (44.5 + 518 + 425.5)$$
$$= 1422.7 \text{ MBq·h}$$

From equation (7),

$$D_{(WB \to WB)} = \tilde{A} \times S_{(WB \to WB)}$$
$$= 1422.7 \times (8.43 \times 10^{-6}) \text{Gy}$$
$$= 0.012 \text{ Gy}$$
$$= 12 \text{ mGy}$$

The maximum total dose to the whole body is now 12 mGy. This is an overestimate of the absorbed dose and is 60% more than that predicted if the second phase is assumed to carry on from 75 hours onwards. It is therefore important to continue performing measurements until the activity in the whole body has fallen to approximately 1% of that injected, if an accurate estimate of the dose is required.

If similar uptakes had been obtained using ^{123}I-mIBG, the effective half-lives would be reduced because of the shorter physical half-life of [123]I. The value of $S_{(WB \to WB)}$ for a 5-year-old for ^{123}I is 2.52×10^{-6} Gy/MBq·h, which is also smaller than that for [131]I. Assuming the second phase of the clearance continues, the whole-body to whole-body dose from 37 MBq of ^{123}I-mIBG would be 0.96 mGy, which is 13% of the ^{131}I dose above.

[123]I is the optimum choice for diagnostic purposes, as it results in the greatest diagnostic information with the lowest possible absorbed radiation dose to the tissues of the patient.

Dose Received During Therapy

The methods for calculating absorbed doses from therapy activities of ^{131}I-labelled mIBG are identical to those used when diagnostic amounts of the radiopharmaceutical are injected. Large activities have been used for targetted radiotherapy with mIBG (typically 3–14 GBq).

Dosimetry of critical organs

In mIBG targetted radiotherapy, there is some radiation risk to all organs that take up mIBG, and therefore it is important to perform dosimetry calculations to assess these risks.

Bone marrow aplasia is the dose-limiting toxic effect of targetted radiotherapy with mIBG, and therefore it would be advantageous to know the potential dose delivered to the bone marrow by a known activity of mIBG. Calculation of absorbed dose in bone marrow is difficult, but an indication of bone marrow dose may be obtained from the estimation of whole-body to whole-body dose, which is much easier to assess (as described above). Reported values of whole-body doses from therapy activities of ^{131}I-mIBG are 0.05–0.3 mGy/MBq (0.37–2.2 Gy from 7.4 GBq), as shown in Fig. 6.5.

The main path of excretion of the mIBG is via the kidneys, and therefore the absorbed dose to the bladder wall from activity in the bladder should be considered. A simple model can be used to estimate this dose. From values of the percentage of injected activity present in each micturition, the mean residence time of the urine in the bladder (taken to be half of the time between successive voids) and the S-values quoted for bladder contents to bladder wall (MIRD 1975b; NCRP 1983), the absorbed dose to the bladder wall can be estimated. Using data from a 9-year-old boy who received 7.4 GBq of ^{131}I-mIBG, and who voided approximately every 5 hours, an absorbed dose of 26 Gy to the bladder wall was estimated. This radiation dose is significant but will vary greatly with the frequency of voiding. It is recommended that continent patients undergoing ^{131}I-mIBG therapy should receive hydration (either oral or intravenous) at a rate of 3 litres per square metre of body surface area per 24 hours for the first 48 hours after administration of the radio-

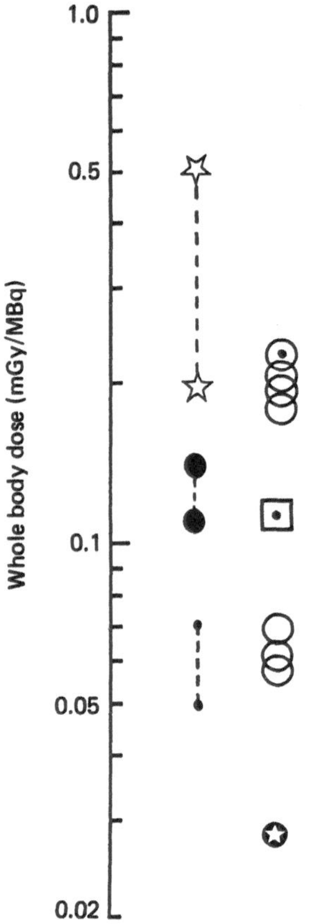

Fig. 6.5. Graph showing published data on whole-body doses per unit activity of ^{131}I-mIBG administered

Symbol	Activity	Disease	Authors
✩	Diagnostic	Neuroblastoma	Lashford et al. 1987
●	Therapy	Phaeochromocytoma	Fischer 1986
·	Therapy	Phaeochromocytoma	McDougall 1984
⊙	Diag/ther	Controls	Amersham Int. 1986
○	Therapy	Neuroblastoma	Hinton et al. 1987
⊡	Diagnostic	Phaeochromocytoma	Ertl et al. 1987
✪	Diagnostic	Animals	Swanson et al. 1981

pharmaceutical, and they should also be encouraged to empty their bladder frequently. Very young or incontinent patients should receive similar hydration, but catheterisation should be considered in order to decrease residence time in the bladder, and to prevent radiation contamination problems associated with urine spills. These precautions will minimise the dose to the bladder wall and to other parts of the urinary tract.

Other organs with relatively high uptake of mIBG are the liver, and the salivary and parotid glands. The absorbed dose to these organs can be calculated using the methods already outlined. Typical values of liver doses from therapy activities of ^{131}I-mIBG are 0.1–1.5 mGy/MBq (0.74–11.1 Gy from 7.4 GBq). Published data on the doses received by a range of organs are shown in Fig. 6.6.

Calculation of tumour dose

The absorbed dose per unit cumulated activity (S-value) for tumours will depend on the position and the size of the tumour. To calculate the absorbed dose in a tumour, it is necessary to go back to first principles and use equation (1). The calculation of absorbed dose in tumours is difficult and subject to error if the tumour is small and the uptake low. The anatomical volume of the tumour can be determined by CT scan or ultrasound measurements, but this volume may differ from the functional volume. Published data on the doses to phaeochromocytomas and to neuroblastomas are shown in Fig. 6.7. In some cases, tumour doses greater than 20 mGy/MBq have been achieved (e.g. 150 Gy from 7.4 GBq).

In view of the difficulties in calculating the absorbed dose to the tumour, the activity to be administered should be chosen to limit the absorbed dose to critical organs (e.g. bone marrow, liver, bladder) to an acceptable level. This can be done by performing a diagnostic, dosimetry study prior to therapy to determine whether the tumour takes up mIBG, and to estimate doses to critical organs.

Using the data shown in Fig. 6.2 as an example, the whole-body to whole-body dose was calculated to be 0.20 mGy/MBq for this diagnostic study. This suggests that 5.0 GBq of ^{131}I-mIBG could be administered to limit the whole-body to whole-body dose (a simple estimate of bone marrow dose) to 1 Gy.

Summary

The basic principles of dosimetry have been outlined, with particular reference to the methods used for the calculation of absorbed doses from radio-iodine-labelled mIBG. An example of the calculation of absorbed dose to the whole body from activity in the whole body has been given. Published

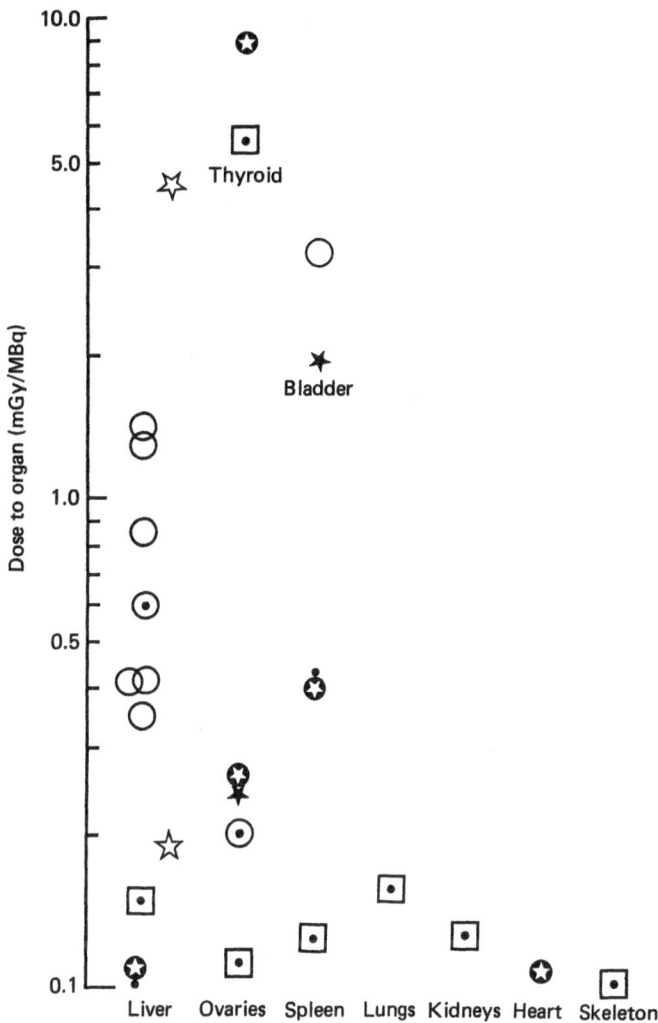

Fig. 6.6. Graph showing published data on doses per unit activity to some organs from ^{131}I-mIBG administered

Symbol	Activity	Disease	Authors
✩	Diagnostic	Neuroblastoma	Lashford et al. 1987
·	Therapy	Phaeochromocytoma	McDougall 1984
⊙	Diag/ther	Controls	Amersham Int. 1986
○	Therapy	Neuroblastoma	Hinton et al. 1987
⊡	Diagnostic	Phaeochromocytoma	Ertl et al. 1987
✪	Diagnostic	Animals	Swanson et al. 1981
✶	Diagnostic	Phaeochromocytoma	Troncone et al. 1984

147

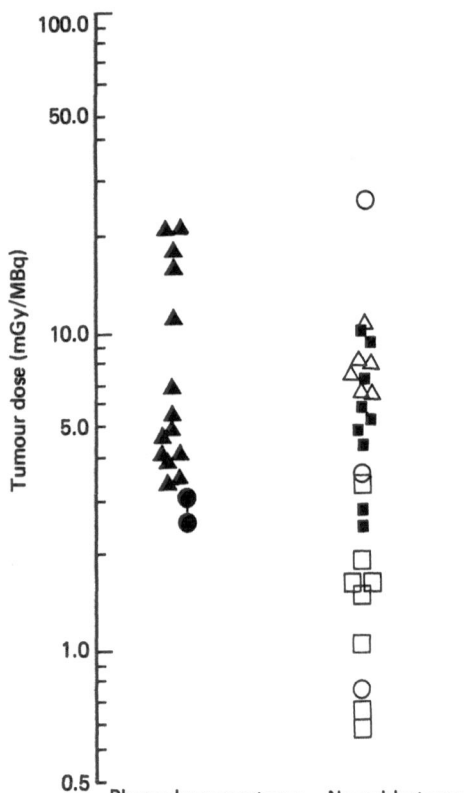

Fig. 6.7. Graph showing published data on absorbed doses per unit activity in phaeochromocytomas and neuroblastomas from therapy activities of ^{131}I-mIBG

▲ Sisson et al. 1984
● Fischer 1986
○ Hinton et al. 1987
△ Feine et al. 1986
■ Schwabe et al. 1987
□ Matthay et al. 1987

data on dosimetry of mIBG has been reviewed and summarised for whole-body doses, organ doses and tumour doses. The accuracy of the dosimetry calculations for radio-iodine-labelled mIBG will depend on the accuracy of calculated activities in organs at various times, the time course considered and the S-values used for the organs of small children.

References

Amersham International (1986) Pack leaflet distributed with diagnostic and therapeutic activities of ^{131}I-mIBG (IBS.6711 and IBS.6712)

ARSAC – Administration of Radioactive Substances Advisory Committee (1988) Notes for guidance on the administration of radioactive substances to persons for purposes of diagnosis, treatment or research, 1 July 1988, p 26

Clarke LP, Malone JF, Casey M (1982) Quantitative measurement of activity in small sources containing medium energy radionuclides: comparison of the gamma camera and rectilinear scanner. Br J Radiol 55:125–133

Ertl S, Deckart H, Blottner A et al. (1987) Radiopharmacokinetics and radiation absorbed dose calculations from ^{131}I-meta-iodobenzylguanidine (^{131}I-mIBG). Nucl Med Commun 8:643–653

Feine U, Klingebiel T, Treuner J (1986) Therapy of the neuroblastoma with ^{131}I-mIBG. In: Winkler C (ed) Nuclear medicine in clinical oncology: current status and future aspects. Springer-Verlag, Berlin, Heidelberg, New York, pp 321–326

Fischer M (1986) Present state of the ^{131}I-mIBG therapy. In: Schubiger PA, Hasler PH (eds) Radionuclides for therapy. Proceedings of 4th Bottsein colloquium, 13–14 June 1986, pp 216–225

Fleming JS (1979) A technique for the absolute measurement of activity using a gamma camera and a computer. Phys Med Biol 24:176–180

Hinton PJ, Fielding SL, Moyes JSE et al. (1987) Quantitative dosimetry for diagnostic and therapeutic ^{131}I-mIBG in neuroblastoma. Nucl Med 26:177

Kereiakes JG, Wellman HN, Simmons G et al. (1972) Radiopharmaceutical dosimetry in pediatrics. Semin Nucl Med 2:316

Lashford LS, Moyes JSE, Ott R et al. (1987) The biodistribution and pharmacokinetics of meta-iodobenzylguanidine in childhood neuroblastoma. Eur J Nucl Med 13:574–577

McDougall IR (1984) Malignant pheochromocytoma treated by ^{131}I-mIBG. J Nucl Med 25:249–251

Matthay KK, Engelstad BL, Huberty JP et al. (1987) Efficacy and safety of ^{131}I-meta-iodobenzyl-guanidine (mIBG) therapy for patients with refractory neuroblastoma. Children's Hospital of Philadelphia, Fourth Symposium on Neuroblastoma Research. Philadelphia, Pennsylvania, May 14–16, 1987

MIRD – Medical Internal Radiation Dose Committee of the Society of Nuclear Medicine Incorporated (New York)
(1969) Pamphlet No. 5. Absorbed fractions for photon dosimetry
(1975a) Pamphlet No. 10. Radionuclide decay schemes and nuclear parameters for use in radiation-dose estimation
(1975b) Pamphlet No. 11. Absorbed dose per unit cumulated activity for selected radionuclides and organs

Myers MJ, Lavender JP, de Oliveira JB et al. (1981) A simplified method of quantitating organ uptake using a gamma camera. Br J Radiol 54:1062–1067

NCRP – National Council on Radiation Protection and Measurements (1983) Report No. 73. Protection in Nuclear Medicine and Ultrasound diagnostic procedures in children

Paić G (1988) Basic dosimetric quantities. In: Paić G (ed) Ionising radiation: protection and dosimetry. CRC Press, Florida, p 35

Poston JW (1976) The effects of body and organ size on absorbed dose: there is no standard patient. In: Cloutier R, Coffey J, Snyder W, Watson E (eds) Radiopharmaceutical dosimetry symposium. HEW Publication (FDA) 76-8044 (National Technical Information Service, Springfield, Virginia) p 92

Schlesinger T (1978) Dosimetry of internal emitters: a guide to the MIRD technique. In: Brodsky A (ed) Physical science and engineering data. Handbook of radiation measurement and protection. Section A, Vol 1. CRC Press, Cleveland. pp 511–526.

Schwabe D, Sahm St, Gerein V et al. (1987) ^{131}I-metaiodobenzylguanidine therapy of neuroblastoma in childhood. Eur J Pediatr 146:246–250

Sisson JC, Shapiro B, Beierwaltes WH et al. (1984) Radiopharmaceutical treatment of malignant phaeochromocytoma. J Nucl Med 24:197–206

Swanson DP, Carey JE, Brown LE et al. (1981) Human absorbed dose calculations for ^{131}I and ^{123}I-labelled meta-iodobenzylguanidine (mIBG): a potential myocardial and adrenal medulla imaging agent. Proceedings of the Third International Radiopharmaceutical Dosimetry Symposium. Health and Human Services Publication, FDA 81–8166. Rockville, Maryland, pp 213–224

Troncone L, Maini CL, De Rosa G, et al. (1984) Scintigraphic localisation of a disseminated malignant phaeochromocytoma with the use of ^{131}I-meta-iodobenzylguanidine. Eur J Nucl Med 9:429–432.

7 Practical Aspects of Targetted Radiotherapy with mIBG

Judy S. E. Moyes, V. Ralph McCready
and Sue L. Fielding

Advances in the management of neuroblastoma have been made in several different areas over the last few years. Mass screening programmes have been developed for the detection of asymptomatic neuroblastoma in children under 2 years of age. These programmes are based on the measurement of urinary catecholamines. Prognosis has been related to histopathological grading, measurement of substances in serum such as serum ferritin and neuron-specific enolase, and amplification of *n* myc. Specific immunological markers have facilitated the diagnosis of minimal bone marrow disease and made differential diagnosis from other small round-cell tumours more reliable. Modest improvements in survival have been achieved by combinations of newer chemotherapy agents in induction programmes, and high-dose chemotherapy and autologous bone marrow transplantation as consolidation therapy (Appendix B). However, despite these advances, long-term survival remains poor in children over 1 year of age with widespread disease at diagnosis. Four-year disease-free survival in these children is only approximately 30%. New ways of approaching the therapy of neuroblastoma therefore clearly need to be devised in an attempt to improve the cure rates. Targetted radiotherapy with mIBG provides one such approach.

General Principles

Targetted radiotherapy using unsealed sources of radiation has been available since the 1940s; however, many questions are still outstanding. In order to eradicate a tumour and for the patient to survive, a high absorbed dose of radiation must be given to the tumour with a minimal dose to the normal tissues. To date, the only successful use of an unsealed radionuclide for therapeutic purposes has been confined to ^{131}I in the treatment of thyroid carcinoma.

The protocols which have been employed for the use of this radionuclide are usually empirical. One method has been to give an initial activity of 3000 MBq (81 mCi) to ablate normal thyroid remnants, followed by subsequent treatment activities of 5550 MBq (150 mCi) to eradicate the differentiated thyroid carcinoma. Successive therapy activities of radio-iodine are given until the lesion is no longer visible on a radioisotope scintigram. However, because it is difficult to accurately measure the functioning volume of tumour it has not been possible to calculate the *actual* radiation dose being given to the lesion and thus discover the dose response of targetted radiotherapy in this disease.

In practice, the level of absorbed radiation dose achieved by a tumour does not always correlate with its response to mIBG therapy. Tumours with apparently high uptake may show poor response, whilst tumours with low uptake may show very good response. This is probably due to a variety of factors, including the heterogeneity of the tumours, the variation in sensitivity of the imaging systems, and the variation of differentiation within the tumour. In the case of adults with differentiated thyroid carcinoma, these details are relatively less important since radioiodine that is not concentrated in the thyroid is rapidly excreted through the gastrointestinal tract and the kidneys. In contrast, however, for the child with neuroblastoma, it is important to estimate more accurately the dose received by the tumour and the whole body, since radiolabelled mIBG is also taken up by the vital organs in addition to the tumour; resulting in side effects, the most significant of which is bone marrow aplasia.

Principles of Therapy with mIBG

The ideal physical and biological properties of a radiopharmaceutical intended for therapy should be such that a large absorbed dose of radiation is received by the tumour with little or no dose to other tissues of the body. In general, radionuclides for therapy are chosen for their abundance of non-penetrating radiations (soft x and γ rays, α, β^-, β^+, internal conversion and Auger electrons), and their lack of penetrating radiations (energetic x and γ rays). In this way, the radioisotope taken up by the tumour emits large quantities of non-penetrating radiations which deposit their energy in a very short tract, so that small tumours can be successfully treated.

In the case of mIBG, suitable isotopes of iodine are ^{131}I, ^{125}I and ^{124}I. ^{131}I has a half-life of 8 days and the most abundant of its wide range of β^- emissions has a mean energy of 192 keV. ^{125}I emits low-energy γ rays, as well as Auger electrons with mean energies of 1–30 keV; ^{124}I is mainly a β^+ emitter. ^{125}I-mIBG may be a useful therapeutic agent in the future: it has a long half-life of 60.2 days, and if the ^{125}I-mIBG is taken up adjacent to or in the cell nucleus, the very short path Auger electrons emitted may give a therapeutic effect limited to that cell over a longer time, sparing surrounding normal cells. Therapeutic activities of ^{124}I-mIBG would be very expensive but the radiopharmaceutical may prove useful, delivering a high dose-rate over a shorter period of time (^{124}I has a half-life of 4.2 days). At present only ^{131}I-mIBG is used regularly for targetted radiotherapy in neuroblastoma, although ^{125}I-mIBG has been used in a few centres. The relatively high-energy γ emissions of ^{131}I are one of the reasons why it is not ideal for targetted radiotherapy, but these do facilitate imaging and dosimetry.

To gain maximum information from therapeutic mIBG, scintigraphic imaging of the patient after administration of the therapy activity should include techniques which can be used for the calculation of absorbed doses to normal tissues and to tumour. This will allow the derivation of optimum activities for administration to minimise damage to normal tissues, and the calculation of a tumour dose-response curve. The methods used for dosimetry estimation of radioiodine-labelled mIBG are outlined in Chapter 6.

Selection of Patients for mIBG Therapy

Many centres are using many different criteria for selection of patients for treatment with radiolabelled mIBG. In some, mIBG is reserved for those children who have failed all conventional treatment. In others it is used for those children who have minimal residual disease, whilst in yet others it is used early on in the course of treatment of their disease. In some centres it is used as a single agent, whilst in others it is used in combination with other treatment modalities. In all centres the patients who are offered mIBG therapy are very carefully selected.

Patients who are expected to survive for less than two months should not be offered this treatment, unless it is being given for palliative purposes (in which case smaller activities should be considered). Patients who are acutely ill, requiring constant or frequent close-contact nursing, medical and parental care, should likewise not be offered this treatment, due to the radiation protection problems which would be encountered. Children whose bone marrow is heavily infiltrated with neuroblastoma, and who on mIBG scintigraphy show increased activity in the bone marrow, should not be offered mIBG therapy since bone marrow aplasia is a well-recognised side effect in these situations. Children with known disease which does not image with tracer activities of radiolabelled mIBG are not eligible for therapy in some centres in the United Kingdom.

The patients who are selected for mIBG therapy must satisfy certain basic criteria: namely, that informed consent is able to be given either by the patient or parents, and that they and/or their families are able to act in a responsible manner towards the inherent hazards of radiation using an unsealed source.

The mIBG Therapy Room

In the United Kingdom, activities up to 11 GBq of ^{131}I-mIBG have been used for therapy purposes, and therefore the intended location of where the therapy will take place has important radiation protection implications. Firstly, these children should be treated in a single room with private toilet facilities en suite. Secondly, they should be treated in a children's unit if possible, since the children will feel more at ease with nurses who are familiar with children. However, in many institutions, the benefits of having paediatric nurses must be weighed up against the benefits of care in an adult unit by nurses who are experienced with the care of patients being treated with unsealed sources of radiation.

The room which is to be designated the mIBG therapy room must comply with local radiation protection guidelines, and therefore structural alterations may be necessary. The room must be protected, with sufficient shielding in the walls, floor and ceiling, to reduce the exposure rate in adjacent rooms to a suitable level. The controlled radiation area (i.e. exposure rates greater than 7.5 μGy/h in the United Kingdom) should not extend further than the therapy room itself.

Large quantities of solid and liquid waste will be produced, and facilities must be available for their safe disposal. If previously designated iodine-therapy rooms are used, then a protected and monitored sewage system may already be in place. If children who are not toilet-trained are to undergo therapy with mIBG, the safe handling of their excreta must be ensured. Catheterisation of these children, with the urinary drainage bag being located in a shielded lead pot, has proved to be an efficient, safe and effective solution to part of this problem. Disposable nappies should also be worn by these children, since these may be disposed of with relative ease should they become soiled with stool.

Facilities should also be available for the parents to be close to their child whilst he or she is being treated. This is very important since in some insti-

tutions most of the non-medical care that the child needs will be provided by the parents, thus reducing to a minimum the exposure to radiation of the medical and nursing staff. Since it is unlikely that any individual child will be involved in more than a limited number of therapies, the parents will therefore be exposed to a limited amount of radiation. The indigenous staff of the therapy unit, however, will potentially be exposed to radiation from a large number of therapies and therefore all possible means of reducing their exposure should be employed. The room available for the parents must also be adequately shielded.

Figure 7.1 shows the floor plan of a single room on a children's unit before conversion for use as an mIBG therapy room. Figure 7.2 shows the same room after it has been converted for use specifically for mIBG therapies. The walls have been reinforced up to a vertical level of 5 feet and lead sheeting has been placed under the bed. Access to the room from the corridor is controlled via the ante-room and via the toilet facilities (both of which can be secured from the inside). The ante-room is used for storage of all items of medical equipment which may be needed during the therapy, for a work-space for nursing and medical personnel and for the location of various radiation detection and monitoring devices. The numbers in the floor plan refer to the exposure rates in μGy per hour at various locations, after a therapeutic activity of 7.4 GBq ^{131}I-mIBG has been given.

Patient Investigations Before Treatment

Different centres will have different protocols for investigation but they should include the following:

1. Full history and clinical examination of the patient.
2. Accurate assessment of the size of the tumour(s) using ultrasound, CT scans, and/or magnetic resonance imaging (MRI).
3. Accurate assessment of the extent of disease using a combination of radiological, histological and biochemical techniques.
4. Dosimetry estimation by mIBG scintigraphy (for example, as described in Chapter 6) to determine the activity of ^{131}I-mIBG to be administered for therapy.

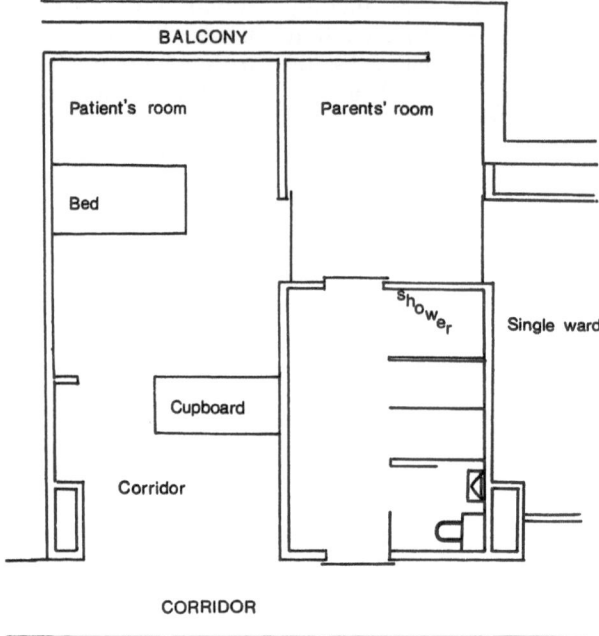

Fig. 7.1. Unmodified single room on a children's ward

5. Baseline haematological and biochemical investigations to monitor bone marrow function, thyroid function, liver function, adrenal function, renal function and electrolyte imbalance.

Drugs which Interfere with mIBG Uptake

Appendix E lists the medicines and over-the-counter preparations which are known, or thought, to interfere with the uptake of mIBG by neuroblastoma. The patient should be asked to avoid these for a minimum of two weeks prior to the projected date of mIBG therapy.

Thyroid Blockade

In-vivo de-iodination of radiolabelled mIBG results in possible uptake of radioiodine by the thyroid gland. The thyroid must therefore be blocked by prior administration of an appropriate medication.

Further details regarding suggested medications are given in Appendix D. Whichever agent is chosen, blockade should start 48 hours before, and continued for two weeks after, the mIBG is administered.

Selection of the Activity of mIBG to Administer

The activity of mIBG to be administered to each patient varies from institution to institution, and the factors which determine the selection of that activity will vary likewise. In some institutions an activity has been selected empirically, and all patients are given the same activity; the response of various tumours and the side effects resulting are then related to that known activity. In other institutions dosimetry estimation studies are performed and an attempt is made to determine an activity which will result in a certain radiation absorbed dose to the tumour, and that activity is given. In yet others, dosimetry estimation studies are performed and from these whole-body radiation doses are determined, the activity of mIBG to be

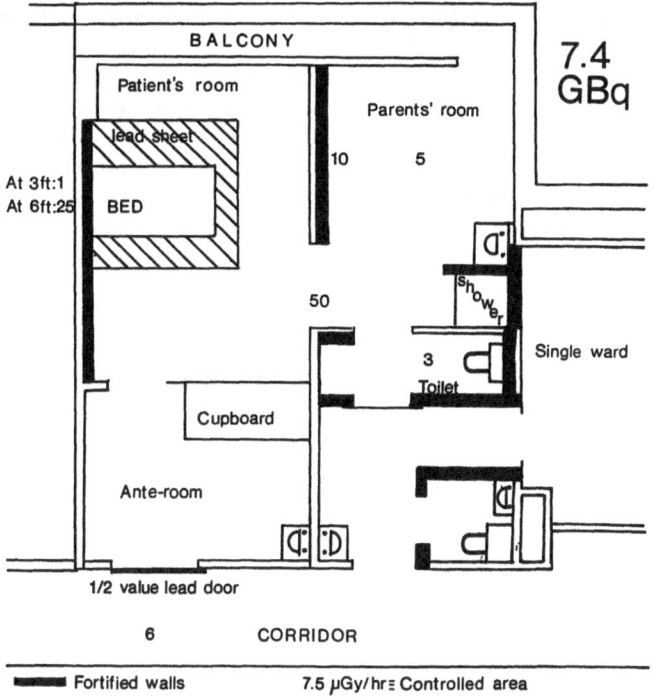

Fig. 7.2. Purpose-adapted single room on a children's ward. This room is the same as that illustrated in Fig. 7.1, but it has been modified by the construction of fortified walls, the addition of a lead-lined door, and lead sheeting to the floor beneath and around the bed. The walls have been screened to a height of 5 feet. The numbers in the diagram represent the dose rates obtained in µGy per hour at several different locations in and around the room, after a therapeutic activity of 7.4 GBq ^{131}I-mIBG had been given (7.5 µGy per hour represents a controlled area in the United Kingdom)

administered being dependent on that which will produce a whole-body radiation dose below a certain predetermined level. These are just a few of the methods currently in use to determine the activity of mIBG to be administered.

The most important point regarding selection of activity is that at present there is no perfect method of selection. Therefore whilst mIBG therapy remains a new and relatively unchartered territory, the selection of the activity should be chosen with patient benefit being the ultimate objective, whilst the constraints of available local facilities and resources which might affect the quantity that can safely be administered are borne in mind.

Sedation of Patients During Therapy

Children over the age of three years are likely to be less emotionally dependent on prolonged episodes of close physical contact with their parents. These children can usually be treated with their parents close by (i.e. within visual and verbal contact) and can be persuaded to stay in their rooms for the duration of the treatment (up to 7–10 days). A substantial amount of pre-treatment organisation and preparation needs to have taken place for these children, in order to ensure that they have plenty of things available within the room to keep them occupied for this period of time. Televisions, videos, personal tape recorders, books and games are useful here.

Children under the age of three, those children who are emotionally dependent on prolonged periods of cuddling, and those children who are thought to be unable to comply with, or tolerate, some of the constraints which are necessarily placed upon them during this type of treatment, may be considered candidates for some form of sedation during the therapy. Light sedation during the first 48–72 hours after administration of the radio-labelled mIBG, when the radiation levels are at their highest, will reduce tension and anxiety quite considerably in some of these situations. The form of sedation chosen will depend on regional variations both in terms of medicines available, and the preferences of affiliated anaesthetists.

Practical Considerations During Administration of mIBG

Administration equipment

The therapeutic activity to be administered may be contained within several vials, and should be drawn up from each of the vials into a single large syringe. That syringe should then be placed onto a shielded battery-driven syringe pump. If the activity is drawn up into several smaller syringes, an unnecessary extra handling dose will be received during syringe exchange at the pump. The syringe pump used for the administration will vary from centre to centre, but it should satisfy the following criteria. It should be easy to load, compact, have simple controls, be able to stand in a horizontal or vertical position, have a loud alarm for indicating malfunction, and a simple on/off switch. It should also have the capacity to provide a wide range of flow rates, and should be encased within purpose-built lead-shielding. The shielding should be constructed in such a way that easy access to the syringe and the controls is possible. Efficient and effective shielding can be achieved by the use of lead bricks, which can be built up around a variety of infusion pumps of different shapes and sizes.

The radiolabelled mIBG should be infused into a good venous line (central or peripheral), and prior to infusion the connections on the venous access route should be checked for leakage.

The length of time taken for the administration of the mIBG will also vary from centre to centre, with times of 20 minutes to 24 hours being reported. The therapy activities of radiolabelled mIBG are usually delivered frozen, therefore thawing must occur before administration. The stability of the thawed radiolabelled mIBG at room temperature will determine the longest possible time over which it may be infused.

Emergency drugs trolley

Theoretically, an anaphylactic reaction or hypertensive crisis may occur during administration of the mIBG, and therefore an emergency drugs trolley containing the necessary medicines for dealing with these situations should be readily available.

Patient-monitoring equipment

Since physical contact with the patient will be limited during an mIBG therapy, equipment for automatic monitoring of the patient's pulse and blood pressure should be available. A visual display of these readings is also necessary.

Fluid requirements

Radiolabelled mIBG is excreted via the kidney and urinary tract. Therefore urine that is present in the bladder is a source of radioactivity to the bladder wall. In order to decrease the potential dose to the bladder, patients should be adequately hydrated with either intravenous or oral fluids, and be encouraged to empty their bladder frequently (in infants catheterisation will be necessary). A fluid regimen of 3 litres per square metre of body surface area per 24 hours will provide sufficient hydration.

Radiation Protection Guidelines

The guidelines employed will vary between institutions depending on local regulations. However, there are some general principles which will be common to all.

Pregnant personnel should not be allowed to attend the patient. Unnecessary contact with the patient should be avoided, but routine nursing care may still be performed, while observing the time restrictions imposed. Protective clothing (gowns, gloves and overshoes) should be worn at all times when caring for the patient or entering the patient's room, and any contamination should be monitored.

The patient should be restricted to his/her room for the duration of the therapy (excluding bathroom privileges), and discharged only when it is deemed safe by the local radiation protection supervisors. Visitors to the patient should be restricted to family and close friends; women who are pregnant and children should be prohibited. All visitors should remain outside the treatment room. The treatment room should not be cleaned for the duration of the therapy.

Food trays and the eating utensils used should all be disposable. Soiled linen should be disposed of by the physics department.

No biological samples (blood, urine etc) should be taken without approval from the radiation protection supervisor. Before dispatching the samples to the appropriate laboratories, the radiation level of each sample must first be cleared by that supervisor.

The importance of careful bathroom habits should be emphasised to children who are toilet-trained. All boys should sit on the toilet when they want to pass urine, so that splashes of urine may be avoided. The toilet should be flushed three times after use and thorough hand-washing performed.

Discharge after mIBG Therapy

In the United Kingdom there are general guidelines laid down in the *Guidance notes for the protection of persons against ionising radiations arising from medical and dental use* (NRPB 1988), which advise on the conditions under which patients may be allowed to leave hospital and return home after the administration of radioactive substances. For children receiving ^{131}I-mIBG for therapy, it is advisable to keep them in hospital until they reach the "no restrictions" level of 150 MBq. It is therefore important to monitor the patient regularly to assess when this level of radioactivity is reached. If the young patient has brothers and sisters at home, restrictions and precautions should continue until the activity is reduced to 30 MBq. Upon release from hospital, the patient should be issued with a card with information regarding the treatment, a date when the special radiation safety precautions cease to apply, and the name of an individual to contact if advice is needed. The special precautions undertaken until the 30 MBq level is reached should include avoiding non-essential contact with young children and pregnant women, using separate disposable eating utensils, flushing the toilet twice after use and avoiding mouth to mouth contact by, for example, toothbrushes and drinking glasses.

Reference

NRPB – National Radiological Protection Board (1988) Guidance notes for the protection of persons against ionising radiations arising from medical and dental use, pp 67–59.

Appendices

Appendix A: OPEC Chemotherapy

The following drugs are used, and given over 5 days.

Cyclophosphamide $600\,mg/m^2$ i.v. stat – day 1
Vincristine $1.5\,mg/m^2$ i.v. stat – day 1 (maximum $2.0\,mg$)
Cisplatin $60\,mg/m^2$ i.v. stat – day 2
Etoposide $60\,mg/m^2$ i.v. infusion over 1 hour – days 3, 4, 5.

These drugs are given in combination with prescribed fluids for hydration, and osmotic diuretics. This combination of chemotherapy agents is repeated approximately every 3 weeks, for a predetermined number of courses.

Appendix B: High-Dose Melphalan Followed by Autologous Bone Marrow Rescue

Melphalan is given in the dose range of 140–220 mg/m^2 by slow intravenous injection, after a good hydration and diuresis has been achieved in the patient. This is followed 12–24 hours later by reinfusion of the patient's own bone marrow. Anti-emetics and anticonvulsants are also given.

Appendix C: Sedation for Children Undergoing mIBG Scintigraphy

Different institutions will have their own preferences regarding sedation. The following "cocktail" (known as TDP) has been prepared by the pharmacists at The Royal Marsden Hospital, and has proved effective on many hundreds of occasions.

Trimeprazine   6 mg
Droperidol   600 μg $\Big\}$ per ml
Methadone 3200 μg

Dose: 0.25 ml/kg – given 1 hour before sedation is required.

Other sedatives which may be considered include chlorpromazine and diazepam. Although chlorpromazine theoretically interferes with mIBG uptake by the tumour, this is unlikely to be a major problem.

Appendix D: Thyroid Gland Blockade for mIBG Scintigraphy and Targetted Radiotherapy

All medication for thyroid blockade should start 24–48 hours before administration of the radiolabelled mIBG. For scintigraphy with ^{123}I-mIBG the medication should be continued for 5 days in total, and for 7 days if ^{131}I-mIBG is used. If ^{131}I-mIBG is used for targetted radiotherapy, then the medication should be continued for a minimum of two weeks.

Any of the following regimens may be used. We have found all of them to be successful, and they are all currently in use at The Royal Marsden Hospital in Surrey.

1. Lugol's iodine 0.2 ml by mouth 3 times per day (or as a single once daily dose of 0.6 ml). This tastes unpleasant and therefore may be diluted in the child's favourite drink without altering its efficacy. We have had no trouble in giving this to small babies in a bottle of juice.
2. Potassium iodide tablets 100 mg per day by mouth.
3. Potassium iodate 170 mg per day by mouth.

Appendix E: Drugs which Interfere with mIBG Studies

There are many drugs and compounds which on a theoretical basis could interfere with the concentration of mIBG by neuroblastoma, for example by interfering with the uptake mechanisms or acting as competitive inhibitors. Therefore the discontinuation of these medicines 2–6 weeks before administration of the radiopharmaceutical should be considered if this is clinically possible. The classes of drugs which have interfered with the uptake of mIBG are tricyclic antidepressants and related drugs, some antihypertensives, phenothiazines, amphetamines and particularly some nasal decongestants and cough preparations.

Patients should therefore be provided with a list of medications to avoid if possible for a minimum of two weeks before mIBG scintigraphy (Tables A.1 and A.2).

Table A.1. Medications to avoid: generic names

Amitriptyline	Methylphenidate
Benperidol	Mianserin
Bretylium tosylate	Nortriptyline
Butriptyline	Oxymetazoline
Chlorpromazine	Oxypertine
Desipramine	Pericyazine
Dexamphetamine	Perphenazine
Diethylpropion	Phentermine
Dothiepin	Phenylephrine
Doxepin	Pimozide
Droperidol	Prochlorperazine
Ephedrine	Promazine
Fenfluramine	Protriptyline
Flupenthixol	Pseudoephedrine
Fluphenazine	Sulpiride
Guanethidine	Thioridazine
Haloperidol	Traxodone hydrochloride
Imipramine	Trifluoperazine
Labetalol hydrochloride	Trifluperidol
Lofepramine	Trimipramine
Maprotiline	Viloxazine
Mazindol	Xylometazoline
Methotrimeprazine	Zuclopenthixol

continued

Table A.2. Medications to avoid: brand names

Actified	Minims Phenylephrine
Allegron	Hydrochloride
Anquil	Modecate
Apisate	Moditen
Auralgicin	Molipaxin
Aventyl	Motipress
Benylin	Motival
Betnovate rectal	Neophryn
Bolvidon	Neulactil
Bretylate	Norval
CAM	Nozinan
Clopixol	Orap
Concordin	Otrivine
Congesteze	Otrivine-Antistin
Depixol	Parstelin
Dexedrine	Pavacol-D
Dimotane	Pertofran
Dolmatil	Phenergan
Domical	Phensedyl
Dospan	Pholcomed
Droleptan	Pholtex
Duo-Autohaler	Ponderax
Duromine	Prothiaden
Eskornade	Ritalin
Evadyne	Rynacrom compound
Fentazin	Serenace
Fluanxol	Sinequan
Fortunan	Sparine
Franol	Stelazine
Gamanil	Stemetil
Ganda	Sudafed
Haldol	Surmontil
Hayphryn	Tedral
Iliadin	Tenuate
Integrin	Teronac
Ionamin	Thalamonal
Ismelin	Tofranil
Isopto Frin	Trandate
Largactil	Triperidol
Lentizol	Triptafen (Tryptafen)
Limbitrol	Tryptizol
Ludiomil	Veractil
Medihaler-Duo	Vertigon
Melleril	Vibrocil
	Vivalan

Appendix F: Modified OPEC Chemotherapy

The following drugs are used, and given over 5 days.

Cyclophosphamide 600 mg/m^2 i.v. stat – day 1
Vincristine 1.5 mg/m^2 i.v. stat – day 1 (maximum 2.0 mg)
Cisplatin 100 mg/m^2 i.v. stat – day 2

Etoposide 60 mg/m^2 i.v. infusion over 1 hour – days 3, 4, 5

These drugs are given in combination with prescribed fluids for hydration, and osmotic diuretics. This combination of chemotherapy agents is repeated approximately every 3 weeks, for a pre-determined number of courses.

Subject Index